'In this remarkable work, the author explores ways of conceiving perversions beyond any moral framework. He portrays them as the instrumentalisation of another's subjectivity, serving the boundless pleasure of a self at once devastating and devastated.'

Elisabeth Roudinesco, *Historian (HDR. Université de Paris VII-Diderot), Teacher at the École normale supérieure in Paris, President of Société internationale d'histoire de la psychiatrie et de la psychanalyse, Honorary Committee Member of the International Sandor Ferenczi Network.*

'This fast and furious book turns psychoanalysis inside out by rethinking the so-called perversions. Aristotle, Freud, Lacan, Stoller, Ferenczi, Butler, Sade, Sacher-Masoch and others are brought into dialogue with case studies that are as gripping as they are unsettling. Bold, provocative, and often controversial, it confronts its subject matter with unflinching intensity.'

Patricia Gherovici, *Psychoanalyst, professor at the Pulsion Institute, New York*

Perversions

Perversions: A Contemporary Introduction offers a comprehensive exploration of psychoanalytic theories of perversion, tracing their evolution from Freud through contemporary practice with particular emphasis on Lacanian perspectives and modern understandings of sexuality and gender.

This book provides readers with a thorough understanding of how psychoanalytic thinking on perversions has evolved and modernised. Drawing on decades of clinical expertise, Sergio Benvenuto examines both sadism and masochism while contextualising paraphilias within contemporary cultural and ethical frameworks. Readers will gain practical clinical strategies alongside rigorous theoretical analysis, moving beyond pathologising approaches to embrace nuanced perspectives on behaviours previously considered perverse. The work bridges historical psychoanalytic thought with current clinical applications, offering vital insights for contemporary practice.

Part of the Routledge Introductions to Contemporary Psychoanalysis series, this fascinating volume is designed for psychoanalysts in training and practice, as well as psychiatrists seeking deeper theoretical grounding. Students and researchers in psychiatry, sociology, sexology, philosophy and Gender Studies will find valuable interdisciplinary perspectives and sophisticated understanding of perversion theory and its application in modern therapeutic contexts, making this an indispensable resource for both academic study and clinical practice.

Sergio Benvenuto is a psychoanalyst and researcher in psychology and philosophy at the National Scientific Research Council (CNR) in Rome, Italy. He teaches psychoanalysis at the International Institute of the Psychology of Depth in Kiev, Ukraine, and at the Institute Pulsion in New York. He is the author of *Lacan, Kris and the Psychoanalytic Legacy: The Brain Eater* (2023), *Conversations with Lacan: Seven Lectures for Understanding Lacan* (2019) and *What are Perversions?: Sexuality, Ethics, Psychoanalysis* (2016).

Routledge Introductions to Contemporary Psychoanalysis

Series Editor: Aner Govrin
Executive Editor: Yael Peri Herzovich

Interpersonal Psychoanalysis: A Contemporary Introduction
Anna Maria Loiacono

Psychodynamic and Psychoanalytic Supervision: A Contemporary Introduction
Christine Driver

Couple Relations: A Contemporary Introduction
Mary Morgan

The Oedipus Complex: A Contemporary Introduction
Poul Rohleder

Psychoanalytic Film Theory: A Contemporary Introduction
Ben Tyrer

Thomas Ogden: A Contemporary Introduction
Ofrit Shapira-Berman

Online Psychoanalysis: A Contemporary Introduction
Haim Weinberg

Psychosis: A Contemporary Introduction
Franco De Masi

Free Association: A Contemporary Introduction
Barnaby B. Barratt

Interpretation: A Contemporary Introduction
Aner Govrin

The Negative: A Contemporary Introduction
Rakefet Efrat Holzer

Harry Guntrip: A Contemporary Introduction
Loray Daws

Gender: A Contemporary Introduction
Oren Gozlan

Traumatic Narcissism Theory: A Contemporary Introduction
Daniel Shaw

Philip Bromberg: A Contemporary Introduction
Anthony Bass, Velleda C. Ceccoli

Antisocial Personality Disorder: A Contemporary Introduction
Jessica Yakeley

Pierre Janet: A Contemporary Introduction
Giuseppe Craparo

Psychoanalysis and Religion: A Contemporary Introduction
Tamas Pataki

Perversions: A Contemporary Introduction
Sergio Benvenuto

For more information about this series, please visit: www.routledge.com/Routledge-Introductions-to-Contemporary-Psychoanalysis/book-series/ICP

Perversions

A Contemporary Introduction

Sergio Benvenuto

Routledge
Taylor & Francis Group
LONDON AND NEW YORK

Designed cover image: © Michal Heiman, Asylum 1855–2020, The Sleeper (video, psychoanalytic sofa and Plate 34), exhibition view, Herzliya Museum of Contemporary Art, 2017

First published 2027
by Routledge
4 Park Square, Milton Park, Abingdon, Oxon OX14 4RN

and by Routledge
605 Third Avenue, New York, NY 10158

Routledge is an imprint of the Taylor & Francis Group, an informa business

British Library Cataloguing-in-Publication Data
A catalogue record for this book is available from the British Library

ISBN: 978-1-032-87201-8 (hbk)
ISBN: 978-1-032-85528-8 (pbk)
ISBN: 978-1-003-53138-8 (ebk)

DOI: 10.4324/9781003531388

Typeset in Times New Roman
by Taylor & Francis Books

Contents

Series Editor's Preface

Aner Govrin

Routledge Introductions to Contemporary Psychoanalysis is one of the most prominent psychoanalytic publishing ventures of our day. The series' aim is to become an encyclopaedia of psychoanalysis, with each entry given its own book.

This comprehensive series illuminates the intricate landscape of psychoanalytic theory and practice. In this collection of concise yet illuminating volumes, we delve into the influential figures, groundbreaking concepts, and transformative theories that shape the contemporary psychoanalytic landscape.

At the heart of each volume lies a commitment to clarity, accessibility, and depth. Our expert authors, renowned scholars and practitioners in their respective fields, guide readers through the complexities of psychoanalytic thought with precision and enthusiasm. Whether you are a seasoned psychoanalyst, a student eager to explore the field, or a curious reader seeking insight into the human psyche, our series offers a wealth of knowledge and insight.

Each volume serves as a gateway into a specific aspect of psychoanalytic theory and practice. From the pioneering works of Sigmund Freud to the innovative contributions of modern theorists such as Antonino Ferro and Michael Eigen, our series covers a diverse range of topics, including seminal figures, key concepts, and emerging trends. Whether you are interested in classical psychoanalysis, object relations theory, or the intersection of neuroscience and psychoanalysis, you will find a wealth of resources within our collection.

One of the hallmarks of our series is its interdisciplinary approach. While rooted in psychoanalytic theory, our volumes draw upon insights from psychology, philosophy, sociology, and other disciplines to offer a holistic understanding of the human mind and its complexities.

Each volume in the series is crafted with the reader in mind, balancing scholarly rigour with engaging prose. Whether you are embarking on your journey into psychoanalysis or seeking to deepen your understanding of specific topics, our series provides a clear and comprehensive roadmap.

Moreover, our series is committed to fostering dialogue and debate within the psychoanalytic community. Each volume invites readers to critically engage with the material, encouraging reflection, discussion, and further exploration.

We invite you to join us on this journey of discovery as we explore the ever-evolving landscape of psychoanalysis.

Aner Govrin

Acknowledgement

I thank Emma Gainsforth and Gianmaria Senia for helping me – each in their own way, by refining the English and copy-editing – bring this book to completion.

Notice

I have decided to translate the Lacanian '*grand Autre*', written with an uppercase 'A', with the Latin term *Alter*, with a capital 'A'. This is because in Latin, there are two distinct uses of what in English is referred to as 'other'. *Alter* (feminine *altera*; neuter *alterum*) refers to the other between two, between an 'I' and a 'non-I', we might say, that is, 'other-than-the-subject'. On the other hand, *alius* (feminine *alia*; neuter *alium*) refers to the other as excluded from a list, like when we say 'These two people are very capable, while the others are incompetent'.

Latin uses *alter* to mean the other in an alternative, *alius* to mean any other from the already listed ones. Now, the Lacanian Other is *Alter* or *Alterum* insofar as it is constitutive of the 'I' or 'myself', and indeed, Lacan never speaks of big Others in the plural, but always and only of *one* big Other. What Lacan refers to as 'other' with a lowercase 'o' corresponds specifically to the Latin *alius* – the others that are taken into consideration only after certain others have been emphasised.

This will allow me to recover the A (capital 'a') of the French *Autre*, which, moreover, has important resonances for those with an Anglo-American cultural background, since it evokes the 'scarlet letter A' in the eponymous novella by Nathaniel Hawthorne.

Chapter 1

What Are Perversions?

Do Perversions Exist?

That a book on perversions should begin by questioning whether they exist might strike some as peculiar. Their existence, however, is not a given. Various schools of thought have cast doubt on whether there is such a thing. Furthermore, the very use of the plural term suggests that it is difficult to conceive of perversions as a unified whole. We never speak of 'hysterias' or 'depressions'.

Mainstream psychiatry has replaced the term *perversions* with *paraphilias*, as reflected in the *Diagnostic and Statistical Manual of Mental Disorders* (DSM). Now in its fifth edition,[1] the DSM was developed by American psychiatry, and it is taught as the Esperanto of psychiatry around the world. The other official manual of psychiatry, the ICD, published by the WHO, is quite similar to the DSM.[2]

The term *paraphilias* was introduced by one of the most influential sexologists, John Money. He drew a distinction between *paraphilia* and *normophilia*, and defined the latter as 'a condition of being erotosexually in conformity with the standard as dictated by customary, religious or legal authority'.[3] Paraphilia is understood here simply as a sexual behaviour deviating from the religious, legal, or customary norm in a given society.

The shift undergone by the term 'paraphilia' clearly reflects the need to do away with the derogatory connotation of perversion,

DOI: 10.4324/9781003531388-1

which in psychiatry refers to sexual acts, but in popular discourse is applied to everything that appears wicked, twisted, sordid. 'Perverse' is an insult.

It must be said that even psychoanalysts often confer this broader, derogatory sense of evil on the term 'perversion'. Consequently, Nazi officials who ran extermination camps like Auschwitz, perpetrators of war crimes or brutal murders, etc., are analysed as perverse and as sadists, in particular. In this volume, we will focus instead on perversions understood as sexual gratifications that are considered 'weird'.

This means that a Nazi death camp commander who performs his duties bureaucratically – for example, Adolf Eichmann – is a monster, but cannot be labelled perverse. However, if such a commander particularly enjoys killing large numbers of people, then he is perverse. What defines perversion is always a distinctive *enjoyment* of some kind, which psychoanalysis has interpreted as sexual in nature. Perversions are forms of sexual enjoyment.

In Greek, *paraphilia* means *loving the wrong things*, just as *paranoia* means believing the wrong things. But even this reference to a *para*, to the strange or wrong, tends to be dropped in more libertarian elaborations. Authentically perverse individuals today would then simply be those whose actions are ethically unacceptable and subject to criminal prosecution, such as paedophiles or sadists. In this context, the ethical-legal assessment becomes the only meaningful feature of perversions. In sum, on the one hand, there are those who commit sexual offences, and, on the other, there is everyone else, from straight heterosexual couples to men who derive pleasure from another man urinating into their mouth.

For psychoanalysis, as we shall see, the same person can adopt either a sadistic or a masochistic position, depending on the circumstances. By contrast, philosopher Gilles Deleuze[4] drew a radical distinction between masochism and sadism, rejecting the concept of *sadomasochism* that had been successful for a very long time. The Deleuzians of today give this distinction a primarily ethical-legal meaning: masochists, they claim, are harmless individuals who enjoy playing games, while sadists are mostly criminals and must be punished. In this way, *perverse* retains the heavily moral connotation it has always borne and which led to the substitution of the term with 'paraphilia'.

In short, 'perversion' remains fundamentally a moral judgement. And, like any moral judgement concerning sexuality, it varies according to the customs and culture of the age.

Today, some of my maso-fetishistic analysands – masochism and fetishism often overlap – classify their practices as a legitimate 'sexual orientation'. (I use the term 'analysands' rather than 'patients' because I do not consider psychoanalysis a medical practice.) The reference here is to LGBTQ+. However, I note that, as far as I know, a 'P' – whether for Perverse or Paraphilic – has not yet been added to this open list. Is this exclusion motivated by the fact that perversion remains a negative attribute even within the LGBTQ+ movement? Or is it because the very concept of perversion or paraphilia is rejected?

In any event, simply dedicating a book to perversions can be seen as a conservative provocation. A legitimate operation would be *to deconstruct* the medical-psychological concept of perversion. However, this is not the path we will take here.

'Of Perversions, This is the Catalogue …'

In this work, I will therefore attempt

(1) to understand what is meant by perversions,
(2) to understand whether perversions as we conceive of them exist,
(3) and consequently, if they do exist, to understand why they do.

The concept of perversion was elaborated by 19th-century positivist sexology, and is therefore just over a century old.[5] The work of the pioneer on the subject, Richard Krafft-Ebing, was motivated by an ethical and judicial mission: to distinguish between libertines and perverts.[6] The former were 'normal subjects' to be judged according to moral criteria and to the criminal laws of the time; the latter were psychiatric patients. If a sexologist had proved that Oscar Wilde's homosexuality was merely a *psychopathia sexualis*, the author would not have been sentenced to hard labour in 1895. At the time, Krafft-Ebing classified homosexuality as a perversion, something that would be unacceptable today, but which, for him, was a way of decriminalising it.

Today's mainstream psychiatry has abandoned the distinction between perverts and libertines, no less because 'libertinism' is no longer considered a crime punishable by law. But DSM psychiatry continues to consider paraphilias *disorders*, and this comes into conflict with a certain queer or woke line of thinking. This perspective argues that psychoanalysts have uncritically adopted the term *perversion* from 19th century sexology without even suggesting an alternative, revealing their complicity with the 'moral epistemology' of old psychiatry. It also points out that many psychoanalysts, especially in America, have in the past supported a psychopathological approach to homosexuality and advocated its treatment. According to this view, psychoanalysts played a role in curbing the revolution in sexual behaviours.

At this point, it is worth looking at what the DSM teaches new generations of psychiatrists on the subject of paraphilias. First, it is worth noting that the manual in question has long favoured the term mental *disorders* over alternatives such as *ailments, diseases*, or *illnesses* – an indication of its efforts to de-medicalise psychiatry. The DSM is structured as a tool designed to standardise the classification of mental abnormalities, primarily through the codification of each disorder using letters and numbers, which can then be managed by computer programmes.

Also worth noting is the fact that the list of paraphilias in the DSM is not very different from that of the pioneers of the psychiatrisation of perversions in the 19th century. In both we find:

- exhibitionism and voyeurism (scopophilia)
- fetishism,
- *frotteurism* (feeling up, rubbing),
- paedophilia,
- sexual masochism and sadism.

The DSM-5 adds a very brief list of 'not otherwise specified' paraphilias: telephone scatologia (obscene phone calls to women), necrophilia (sexual acts involving corpses), partialism (in the DSM-IV exclusive sexual focus on a specific part of the body other than the genitals), zoophilia (sex with animals), coprophilia (sexual arousal from faeces), klismaphilia (passion for enemas) and urophilia (sexual attraction for urine).

The list of perversions could be endless. Take, for example, *symphorophilia* (from *symphoron*, adversity), coined by Money – the pursuit of sexual arousal through the staging of disasters, such as catastrophic car crashes. A group of car crash paraphiliacs are the protagonists of J. G. Ballard's novel *Crash*.[7]

There is the rare but unsettling *vorarephilia* (or *vore*), an erotic fantasy involving the act of devouring or being devoured by another living person.[8] This differs from sexual cannibalism in that vorarephilia revolves around the fantasy of swallowing someone whole and alive, whereas cannibalism entails the desire to consume or even just cook parts of a person's body.

We have the *macrophilic* (GTS fetish), a fascination with giants, most commonly giant humans, but also giant objects. This attraction often takes an explicit sexual tone. Macrophilists are generally men who imagine themselves dealing with huge women if they are heterosexual, or with huge men if they are homosexual. These giants casually crush and destroy entire cities, like erotic King Kongs. The phantasy can reverse: they imagine themselves as enormous beings crushing small (normal) ones.[9]

All forms of paraphilia are now shared through specialised social networks, and this allows paraphiliacs to connect across the world with like-minded individuals who share their erotic passions. This helps them feel less isolated and less 'monstrous'.

Certain exclusions to the list, which the DSM-5 in particular presents compared to older editions, stand out. Homosexuality is, of course, absent, but so are incest and gerontophilia (sexual attraction of young people to old people). In fact, in the sexology of the past, gerontophiles were mostly men, hardly ever women. Today, however, we have all accepted the romantic principle that 'love knows no age', which precludes modern psychiatry from seeing anything pathological in a relationship between two people with an age gap of 30 years or more.

It is also interesting to note the absence of incest from the catalogue, even though it is a very frequent practice. What makes the psychiatric establishment think that a mother or father who has sex with an adult son or daughter is not a paraphiliac? Incest with underage children falls under paedophilia, of course, but sex between close relatives over the age of consent is presumably not a disorder simply because in the modernised world[10] any sexual relation between consenting adults is no longer considered a punishable act. In fact, the psychiatric framework is not purely 'scientific' in the sense that it is not entirely distinct and independent from the criminological framework.

It cannot be said, however, that psychiatry relies entirely on modern law in the case of incest, since in many countries incest between adults is a criminal offence; but I wonder to what extent it is actually punished in many of these countries. The list of countries that *do not* criminalise incest between adults is much shorter than the list of countries that do, even though the former do not allow marriage between close blood relatives. A prominent example of countries where incest is a criminal offence is the United Kingdom and the former British colonies. Incest is not an offence in China, but it is in Hong Kong, precisely because it was under British jurisdiction for over a century. Otherwise, the laws appear to be distributed quite arbitrarily. In Germany, for example, same-sex incest is legal, while incest between people of the opposite sex is punishable by up to three years in prison; in Switzerland, the opposite is true.

Nevertheless, it seems that in the modernised world the legal systems are moving toward decriminalising incest between consenting adults, and the feeling is that it has remained punishable only on paper as a sediment of an earlier jurisprudence.

One reason for the exclusion of incest from the list of perversions is the growing uncertainty in assessing incestuous relationships, which we have only recently come to recognise as widespread behaviours. This relaxed approach to incest appears in a number of contemporary novels and films.

However, the DSM-5 does not tell us *why* we should consider certain sexual acts to be paraphilias, or *why* they are mental disorders, i.e. phenomena that disrupt an established order.

In Freud's time, the *established order* was heterosexual coitus with the potential for conception. It would be a caricature of this traditional position to claim that only reproductive sex was allowed; if it were true, intercourse with postmenopausal or sterile women would also have been forbidden, which was not the case. The point was that intercourse, even if sterile, had to be enacted *as if* it were fertile. If coitus did not serve to impregnate a woman, may it at least *simulate* the act of doing so.

According to this view, orgasm was the end that justifies the means: anything goes, as long as you and your partner reach orgasm, which centuries ago was called 'the little death'. Dying in pleasure was the goal that made sexual play 'normal'. A common theory in the Middle Ages was that a woman could only become pregnant if she reached orgasm during intercourse in a fertile period. This was linked to Galen's two-seed theory, according to which both man and woman needed orgasm for conception. Female enjoyment was the condition for fertility.[11]

All acts that did not correspond to this simulation of fertile intercourse were therefore labelled perverse, including anal penetration of women, oral sex, homosexual coitus, etc. Until even a few decades ago, kissing and caressing were not considered perverse unless they involved the other's genitals, which could come into contact exclusively with the genitals of the opposite sex. Even the use of hands to touch the partner's genitals was forbidden. As late as the 1960s, for example, even psychoanalysts who were considered to be rather nonconformist referred to cunnilingus and fellatio as perversions.

I would say the opposite is true today: if a woman or man shudders at the thought of oral or anal sex, they would be more likely to be advised to consult a sexologist or a psychologist.

Today, 'perversions' such as oral sex and anal intercourse are enjoyed by a vast portion of the population. The evolution of behaviours has in fact forbidden hegemonic psychiatry to occupy itself with homosexuality, gerontophilia, fellatio, incest, as pathologies … or rather, as disorders.

Most psychoanalysts have conformed to this dominant view, albeit not without some reluctance.

From Aristotle to Utilitarianism

The concept of perversion still seems to be related to what we consider today to be the 'right' or 'wrong' thing to do. Changing the name to *paraphilia* does little to disguise the moral nature of the concept. We shall see in what sense.

Actions are good or bad, normal or pathological, in relation to a *law* or to the basic ethical criteria of a culture. The criterion that inspired positivist psychiatry at the end of the 19th century was basically the same as that of the Christian churches of the time, and is still the criterion followed by conservative opinion today: it was the opposition, derived from Aristotle, between what is *in accordance with nature* and what is *contrary to nature*. In this Aristotelian view, perverse sexuality was considered 'pathological' for the same reasons as homosexuality was: because neither perversions nor homosexuality naturally led to the insemination of women. This opposition between acts 'against nature' and acts 'in accordance with nature' took on a distinctly moral tone, particularly in official Christian morality. In this sense, the *para-* in 'paranoia' and 'paraphilia' can today be understood as meaning *against* in the Aristotelian sense: paranoia is against-the-mind, and perversion is against-love. One must take a stand and *oppose* that which is *against*.

For the philosophy that prevails today, however, the opposition between 'against nature' and 'in accordance with nature' no longer holds. In our age, we believe that everything that exists is natural. Nothing can be against nature because nothing exists outside of nature. Therefore, if we can speak of perverse acts today, it is not because they are supposedly *against nature*, but because they are considered to be *against ethics*. This is due to the fact that in the modernised world, despite the resistance of conservative opinion, the *utilitarian* philosophical conception tends to prevail.

It is impossible to understand the great ethical, legal, political and even psychiatric transformations of the last 70 years without recognising that utilitarian philosophy is the official philosophy of the modernised world. In particular, it explains the broadening of civil rights, which are based on a utilitarian conception. Developed by philosophers such as Hume, Bentham, and Mill, utilitarian theory posits that human beings are governed by two sovereign masters: the pursuit of pleasure and the avoidance of pain. Jeremy Bentham put it very succinctly:

> Nature has placed mankind under the governance of two sovereign masters, *pain* and *pleasure*. It is for them alone to point out what we ought to do, as well as to determine what we shall do. On the one hand the standard of right and wrong, on the other the chain of causes and effects, are fastened to their throne.[12]

Utilitarian ethics is therefore based on the 'pleasure principle', a principle taken up by Freud. This explains why the legal recognition of same-sex marriage is becoming increasingly widespread: since in a homosexual relationship each person gives pleasure to the other, it is a relationship that the state can recognise as a 'good thing'. Utilitarianism truly embodies the hedonistic ideal.

From this perspective, the perverse act is 'a bad thing' – and hence punishable under criminal law – *only if* it causes some actual harm to the other, as in the case of sadism and paedophilia.

The perverse act is considered morally neutral if it causes no obvious harm to others, as in the cases of fetishism, masochism, and transvestism. (Some predominantly Muslim-majority countries, plus Malawi and Uganda, prohibit cross-dressing).

What are the criteria that motivate psychiatry today to classify both 'bad' and 'neutral' sexual acts under the general umbrella of paraphilias? In what sense can we consider even a harmless game – for example, certain masochistic rituals or sex with an animal – to be paraphilic, i.e. *para*, 'bad'?

I think that the criterion that leads a psychiatrist or psychoanalyst to diagnose perversion or paraphilia is indeed ethical. Perversions remain a supposed transgression of sexual ethics, even if often psychiatrists or psychoanalysts may not be aware of it.

Before clarifying in what sense the diagnosis of perversion is 'ethical', we will therefore consider the psychoanalytic theory of perversions.

Freud: From Polymorphous Perversity to Fetishism

There are at least two stages in Freud's approach to perversions.

Initially, he considered perverse all forms of sexuality that did not directly or indirectly aim at coitus. Freud adopted the definition of perversion prevalent in the 19th century, which, as we have seen, referred to sexual acts that deviate from their 'natural' end – namely, the genital satisfaction of an adult.

This is why Freud said that the child is polymorphously *perverse*: the child is not aware of the orgasmic result of sexuality, and so derives sexual pleasure from body parts and objects disconnected from genitality. In short, the child is like a sexual wildcard. In his earlier writings, therefore, perversion appears as a positive, authentic sexuality, not subject to the more refined demands of love for the other and the reproductive task.[13]

But for Freud, as for Wordsworth, 'the child is father to the man',[14] i.e. adult sexuality remains fundamentally infantile. So-called perversions then reveal in men and women an infantile 'perverse polymorphism' that remains the matrix of human sexuality.

Yet, with adolescence young humans confer a hierarchical order to their sexual drives. Adult perversion would then appear to be an overflow of satisfactions unrelated to the genital act in itself. In other words, for Freud perversion was sexuality in its rawest form, not channelled by tenderness for the other or directed towards any orgasmic end; it was an entirely *positive* sexuality unconcerned with the difference between the sexes. It is sexuality as some Dionysian philosophers, such as Deleuze and Guattari,[15] would later celebrate it.

This is the sense of Freud's statement that 'neurosis is the *negative* of perversion'.[16] For him, the neurotic symptom arises from the unconscious staging of a perverse fantasy, whereby what was originally pleasurable – perverse enjoyment – is experienced as ego-dystonic, as unpleasant, as neurotic symptomatology. Neurosis 'negativises' in the sense that it 're-edits' a pleasurable experience as unpleasant. It is as if neurosis muddles and confuses the utilitarian principle, negativising perverse pleasure into unpleasant feelings.

As we shall see, this reversal also occurs in perversions, but in the opposite sense: the *perverse act is mostly the repetition in a pleasurable erotic key of an originally unpleasant trauma.*

Freud later corrected his thesis, which owed much to a myth of the time: perversion as free and uninhibited sexuality. After all, what could be 'positive' or 'natural' about a fetishist who can only get an erection with a woman if she is wearing high heels? More than elsewhere, in perverse eroticism we find a certain sophisticated negativity. When confronted with some specific perverse acts, Freud set aside this 'positive' idea of perversion. In his new approach, instead, what emerges is the centrality of the perversion in its relation to female sexuality, something he had not seen before.

The central text that introduced this later theory of perversion is the paper *Fetishism.*[17] Here Freud sees the sexual fetish as a kind of surrogate penis: fetishistic desire invests the woman as long as … she possesses a penis. The fetish – most often a lady's shoes or feet – as a detachable part or an appendage of the body is like a prosthetic penis. For the non-fetishist man, the female body *evokes* and *invokes* the penis precisely because it lacks one. In fact, heterosexual men are aroused by the shape of the mons Veneris precisely because it emphasises the absence of the penis. Instead, for the fetishist the woman is a source of arousal precisely because of the surrogate penis she displays: for the fetishist, the woman *exhibits* 'her' penis precisely insofar as *she shows it as not belonging to her.* In any case, the tendency of women in many cultures to adorn their bodies with necklaces, earrings, bracelets, etc., reveals a female desire that complements fetishism, the 'female masquerade' as Joan Riviere called it,[18] in which women find pleasure in displaying an artificial phallus – the mask – precisely to enhance their lack of a phallus.

Fetishism reveals a mechanism of negation that Freud calls *Verleugnung*, disavowal: in this case, the disavowal of the lack of a penis in a woman. In the later reworking of the Freudian system, disavowal becomes the specific mode of negation of all perversions. Something at the root of perverse hetero-dystonia, and different from *Verdrängung* (repression), which is at the root of neurotic ego-dystonia.

To systematically illustrate the differences between neurosis, perversion, and psychosis, I will refer to the framework Jacques Lacan developed for these three structures. While this framework was devised by Lacan, it is nonetheless in line with Freud's doctrine.

According to Lacan, neurosis, perversion, and psychosis are not three groups of psychopathologies, but three structures that characterise every human being. Each of us must fall into one of these three forms of negation; there is no fourth possibility. A framework that many, quite rightly, find too restrictive.

If neurosis is based on repression and perversion of disavowal, psychosis results from a form of negation, which Freud does not specify and that Lacan called the *Verwerfung, foreclosure*, of certain privileged, structuring signifiers. Neurotic negation consists essentially in a 'sweeping under the carpet', perverse negation in a 'denial of a lack', and psychotic negation in 'having no access to'.

From this point of view, we can also consider perverse subjects who do not exhibit evident perversions, which opens up the possibility of describing *perverse subjective structures* beyond actualised sexual behaviour. Just as we can describe neurotic structures that do not develop into neurosis in the clinical sense, and psychotic structures without the subject being diagnosed as psychotic. I also believe that analytic theory is still far from being able to describe a pure neurotic, perverse, or psychotic structure.

Even if today many psychoanalysts use a heavily psychiatric language, in which the essential thing seems to be to distinguish the 'pathological' from the 'healthy', I am persuaded that Freudian theory is fundamentally a-psychiatric or even anti-psychiatric. In the sense that psychoanalysis dissolves the very concept of 'psychopathology'. The only thing we can say is that with so-called 'psychopathology' it is always a case of *dystonia. Ego-dystonia* in the case of 'neurosis', *hetero-dystonia* in the case of 'perversions', *socio-dystonia* in the case of 'psychosis'.[19]

This is the pattern that organises the three negations and their effects.

Table 1.1 The Table of the Three Structures

"PSYCHOPATHOLOGY"	*MODE OF NEGATION*
NEUROSIS Phobia Hysteria Obsessional-Compulsive Neurosis	REPRESSION (*Verdrängung*)
PERVERSIONS Fetishism – erotic Masochism Sado-masochism, Sadism, feminine Masochism Voyeurism – Exhibitionism Crossdressing Zoophilia, *frotteurisme*, paedophilia, coprophilia, necrophilia, etc.	DENIAL (*Verleugnung*)
PSYCHOSIS PARANOIAS - Persecution Delusion - Megalomanic Delusion - Erotomania - Jealousy Delusion - Querulomania SCHIZOPHRENIA - Paranoid - Hebephrenic - Catatonic	FORFEITURE, foreclosure (*Verwerfung; forclusion*) of the Name-of-the-Father
OUT OF RANGE BIPOLARITY former MANIC-DEPRESSIVE PSYCHOSIS – Mania and Melancholia AUTISM BORDERLINE personalities PSYCHOPATHY ADDICTIONS Feminine EATING DISORDERS GENDER DYSPHORIA or DYSTONIA – Transgenderism	

The Fetishist's Simulacrum

So, perversions would be based on a specific kind of negation, referred to in English as *disavowal* – sometimes the term *denial* is preferred. Disavowal is evident in the formation of the erotic fetish, as we have seen. The fetish – which becomes the condition for sexual arousal – is therefore the substitute object for the missing female penis. But in what sense is this object a *substitute*?

Very often, perverse disavowal is mistakenly conflated with a denial of reality. But if this were the case, fetishists would be psychotic; they might even hallucinate a penis between a woman's legs, for example, as a result of denying its absence. In fact, *disavowal* – like *Verleugnung* in German – does not mean a pure denial of reality. Dictionaries define *disavowal* as 'the denial of any responsibility in relation to something or someone'. For example, *a husband can disavow his wife*, not in the sense that he denies their marriage, but in the sense that he denies the marital bond with her. We must therefore understand the boy's disavowal of the girl's lack of a penis not as the denial of the non-existence of a female penis, but as a denial of the *value* of that absence. In other words, he accepts the absence of a penis on a perceptual level, but not on the level of desire: *he in no way desires* that the girl lacks a penis.

As an adult, then, the fetishist *desires* the woman, just disavowing her lack of a penis. How is this possible? And how does this disavowal give rise to the fetish, that is, to such an erotically compelling object?

In reality, quite often the fetish is not an object from the woman's actual body; it is not, in other words, a supposed female penis. It is a *signifier*, specifically, the signifier of the lack of a penis, which is quite different. Fetishism, then, is not a denial of reality, but a denial of a signification. Let us see how this takes place.

Disavowal, being a form of negation, implies the symbol 'not'. Human language, in fact, is characterised precisely by the introduction of the 'not' symbol, unlike analogic systems of communication. The 'not', in most languages, has this particularity: it is always *added* to an affirmative sentence in order to negate it. If I say 'Mary wants to eat cherries', I affirm something; if I say

'Mary DOES NOT want to eat cherries', I negate it by inserting a 'does not'. The point is that we must first affirm something in order to deny it. In other words, to signify the absence of something, we must *name* that something in order to express its absence. Absence is always the absence of something – there can be no absence of nothing, because then … nothing is missing. We must always first affirm something, that is, provide the symbol of this thing, in order to negate it. In reality, nothing is ever simply absent; something is always missing in relation to some expectation of it. If I say 'the woman lacks a penis', I mean that a penis was expected and has in fact not been found. The 'not', then, is always subjective; it is 'not' for a subject; it is therefore a purely logical matter, of the logos, not of the thing itself.

To express in an ideographic language that Mary does not wish to eat cherries (which does not necessarily mean she will refuse them), we can depict cherries with a drawing and place a red bar over them, as is commonly done in signs that prohibit certain actions. This also illustrates a general symbolic procedure, for example, a picture of a lit cigarette with a red slash through it means 'No smoking'. In such an ideographic representation, the image of the negated or missing object must be shown, and the slash symbol added to it. Now, let us suppose that Mary does not want to eat the strawberries but instead desires precisely what represents that absence. In other words, she wants the drawn strawberries. In that case, we would have a fetish-object of food desire.

So, we may say that fetishism is not a way of ignoring that women have no penis; it is the desire for the symbol of this negation. The fetishist does not desire the woman to have a penis, unlike the clients of cross-dressing sex workers, for example, as those individuals genuinely desire a woman with a penis – and we do not call them fetishists. The fetishist is fine with the woman having a vagina, but the vagina is not enough for him; he also wants the woman to carry the signifier of the penis precisely as the symbol of its absence. And, as we have seen, the symbol of the absence of something is the signifier or image that represents that missing thing, like the slashed-out image of the cherries. To highlight the negation, I must express the thing being negated and then cancel it as a thing by saying, 'it's only a symbol!' If Mary were to say, 'I want the symbol that negates cherries', this symbol, as we have seen, still represents cherries. Unlike a man who is not perverse, who appreciates in a woman the lack of a penis, the *perverse subject desires the symbol of the lack of a penis.* Therefore, the fetishist desires the symbol of the absence of the penis, which is … an image of a penis. The fetishist seeks the woman insofar as *she is marked by the signifier* of the absence of a penis. Some analysts use the word *phallus* to describe not the missing penis itself, but the *signifier* of its absence.

We may illustrate this with an invented example. Let us imagine that a woman leaves and gives her partner a keepsake to remember her by, like a portrait of herself. Over time, the man falls increasingly in love with that portrait and eventually forgets the real woman. But then the woman returns, and the man goes back to loving her … only if she wears the portrait when they make love. His love for the real woman becomes inseparable from the portrait, which signified her absence.

The effect of the disavowal of the absence of the penis is therefore the investment in a new object: the signifier or *ersatz* of its absence. The classic example of a woman's shoe adored by the fetishist, who perhaps obsessively collects shoes, resembles the penis in that it is an appendage that can be detached from the body (the penis always appears to be detachable). But the resembling fetish-object does not replace the missing real penis; it signifies it. We can now understand why fetishism is often associated with erotic masochism. The masochist is not someone who wants to be subjected to a woman – quite the opposite! He is often a person of high social standing who looks down on ordinary people and is especially eager to dominate women. Why, then, does he stage – the masochistic act is a performance, a play – his degrading submission to a woman? We may say he rather wants the *simulacrum* of submission to the woman. Just as the fetish is a simulacrum of the penis that signifies its absence, similarly the masochistic submission-punishment is the simulation of subjection to the woman. In other words, the masochistic act is the disavowal of a certain feminine impotence, which gives enjoyment insofar as it is precisely a negation of that impotence.

A young man became a masochistic fetishist due to a vivid memory from when he was 4 years old: while playing with his younger brother with a toy gun, he accidentally hit him, not seriously, and their mother reacted furiously by stomping on the toy gun with her blue shoes. This vivid flash memory of the gun being stepped on structured his life. Since then, he can only become sexually aroused when a woman steps on him wearing shoes, especially if the shoes are blue. But the mother's reaction at the time seemed to him more a sign of impotent rage. In adult sexual life, he always had to let the woman 'take it out on him' by being trampled.

In short, the masochist continually denies female subjection … but can only do so by evoking the simulacrum of its opposite. While the fetishist 'gives' the woman a penis in the form of a mock, the masochist 'gives' her great power, but again, in the form of a mock.

And we can see why psychoanalysis tends to view other perversions through the lens of fetishistic disavowal. This is because all perverse acts are simulacrum-acts: the object of pleasure is always the disavowal of something that the woman lacks.

The exhibitionist disavows the fact that the woman rejects the sight of his penis. He stages an act in which it instead appears that the woman is enchanted by this sight. The simulacrum here is the fascinated and desirous gaze of the woman who looks at his penis. The denial of a failure – the woman's utter disinterest in the penis – is represented through its reversal: a woman who desires to look at the male sex.

The object from which the voyeur derives pleasure is not the sight of a woman pleasurably engaged in sexual intercourse – for that, a pornographic film would be enough. The voyeur also takes pleasure in a simulacrum, which inverts the woman's intention not to show her sexual enjoyment. It is *as if* the woman were exhibiting her sexuality in front of others. Also here, the simulacrum is the inverted image of what is disowned: the woman reveals her sexual enjoyment to the subject.

While fetishism and masochism are two ways of returning power to the woman over the man, scopophilias – the perversions of the gaze – are restitutions of the female capacity to enjoy. Perversions are ultimately a way of giving the woman her due in the form of a signifier.

Cross-dressers disavow the fact that men are attracted to the feminine lack of a penis: they actually manifest the fact that men are attracted to feminine beings who have a penis. Of course, in reality this is not the case, but in perversion reality does not matter – signifiers do. So, the cross-dresser enjoys the signifier *woman with phallus* inasmuch as (s)he attracts men. The male fetishist enjoys the signifier of the female phallus; the transvestite, instead, enjoys the attraction that the female phallus exerts over other men. Transvestism is the enjoyment of another person's fetishism.

It is no coincidence that many cross-dressers say that when dressed as women, they feel far more self-confident, energetic, and uninhibited. It is as if their appearing as women in the eyes of others gives them a special phallic power, a virile assertiveness. The signifier of the lack of the phallus gives them a supplementary phallic power.

With the two 'criminal' perversions, sadism and paedophilia, it seems that there is no recourse to simulacra. Here we must make a distinction between a properly sexual sadism and a reactive sadism, and distinguish a platonic paedophilia from a properly perverse one.

The sadist is not someone who takes pleasure in making another person, man or woman, suffer because that person is the object of his contempt or hatred. A person who inflicts harm on a hated enemy is not a sadist in the perverse sense. In fact, the sexual sadist assaults women because he seeks to 'punish' their being-woman, and, above all, to punish *her* pleasure derived from sexual intercourse. In other words, what he aims at in the individual woman is *femininity* itself, and this is a signifier. The sadistic act does not de-sexualise women; it is rather the *staging* of a de-sexualisation.

The paedophile who actively seeks a child can be considered perverse to the extent that he disavows infantile non-genitality. Everyone thinks children are horrified by adult (genital) sexuality, but a paedophile denies this and sometimes even succeeds in seducing a child through tenderness. However, the paedophile also knows that a child is incapable of adult genitality, and thus the paedophilic act is, in fact, a semblance of the child's sexual desire.

The question of fetishism is complicated by the fact that, in the Western (Judaeo-Christian) world, many women seem to regard men's relation to the feminine as essentially fetishistic. We have already spoken of the 'feminine masquerade' as a means of appearing more seductive. Although many women prefer to think that their love of jewellery stems from a kind of solitary self-gratification, analytic practice suggests that, deep down, some of them are convinced that it makes them more seductive to men. In other words, they appeal to a supposed male fetishism – one that is, for the most part, imaginary.

Perhaps the reason for this current male 'fetishism' lies in the fact that the woman presents herself to the male world as a *luxury*. Sexual intercourse can be routine. The woman fears that if this becomes routine for the man, he will cease to love and desire her. In a society where possessing a penis was a sign and condition of power, the woman opposed fetishes to the penis, presenting herself as a precious, rare object, as *something that gives more than what is necessary*. Human sexuality has this strange characteristic: that while it is an ordinary need, it feeds on extraordinariness. Human sexuality demands or dreams of luxury. It is as if women knew that men are attracted to women who are equal to them in phallic stature, even if that stature is provided by clothes and ornaments. Because under a woman's dress, there is no … thing.

This may perhaps shed light on the maso-fetishist, and especially on his 'feminist' inclination, his need to over-qualify the woman, to compensate or avenge her. The woman for the maso-fetishist is not important only for her natural body; she is important as a dominatrix, insofar as she has power over the man. We cannot therefore say with certainty that the fetishist denies female 'castration', as classical theory claims, because he acknowledges a female lack, which in the past was also social and political, and seeks to balance and compensate for it, even if only *in effigy*.

Perversions and Femininity

Freud also reflected on sadomasochistic acts, ascribing to them a meaning that extends far beyond sexual perversions.[20] His reflections on sadomasochism would lead him to identify a profoundly destructive dimension in the human psyche, which may take an extroverted form (sadism) or an introverted one (masochism), but which would appear to him more and more as primary, that is, independent from the dynamics of sexuality and, consequently, of the pleasure principle itself. In short, over time Freud became increasingly interested in the non-utilitarian dimension of human subjectivity, an aspect that his successors would rarely pursue. In other words, what transpires from the enjoyment of sadistic and masochistic acts is a drive that Freud would call the 'death drive' (*Todestrieb*), insofar as it completely escapes the logic of individual satisfaction, i.e. the principle of utility.[21] We can say that in time Freud would develop a theory in which utilitarianism somehow refutes itself.

In this case sadism and masochism lose their perverse specificity in order to become something *beyond* the pleasure-desire principle. The death drive, which expresses itself in masochistic and sadistic destructivity, is beyond any analytic interpretation and represents the limit of any psychoanalytic reconstruction.

But how does Freud explain the specifically male feature of perversions? He does not, but we can grasp his fundamental thought on the matter. In a sense, he believes that women do not indulge in perversions because all femininity is ultimately a perversion, if it is a successful femininity. 'Successful' women are basically masochistic. The question arises about what is meant by 'successful femininity', which can be opposed to hysteria in particular as a failed femininity. 'Successful' for a woman probably means accepting to play a feminine role in sexual intercourse with men, in the sense of deriving pleasure from them and reaching orgasm. Whereas the hysteric is a woman who identifies with a male role.

But what about lesbian sexuality? Are there 'successful' and 'unsuccessful' lesbians?[22] The question remains open.

Today's feminist thinking rejects this Freudian view, but in fact Freud actually attributes to female sexuality a sophistication that male sexuality lacks. For Freud, women are sexually masochistic, and they find enjoyment in that. But perversion – even masochistic – is in a way a sophisticated version of sexuality in men.

Female masochism is primarily expressed through fantasies that many women act out in sex games. We don't label as 'disordered' women who want to be insulted by a man during intercourse, whereas if a man were to ask his partner to insult and humiliate him, he would immediately be branded as 'paraphilic'. Some women enjoy the phantasy of being stopped in the street and raped by a stranger, of being part of a harem, or of being chosen among other women in an old-fashioned brothel. Along these lines, we can go as far as fantasies like those described in *Histoire d'O*, Pauline Réage's famous pornographic novel[23] about the voluntary enslavement of a woman to a man's will. We do not typically find such fantasies in a 'normal' man; on the contrary, the man often likes to play along by insulting the partner who wants to be insulted. This is why, at the height of coitus, a man may ask a woman 'You like it, don't you, bitch?', while some women may say to the man 'Have fun fucking … me!' 'Don't stop!' She enjoys feeling like an object of the man's amusement.[24]

Some will argue that this difference in behaviour is a product of the 'patriarchal' division of genders, according to which it is seen as 'normal' for a woman to submit to a man as an object of contempt, whereas if a man submits to a woman in order to be humiliated, it strikes us as morbid masochism. This is partly true. But it is also true that it is more difficult for the human female to adapt to heterosexual intercourse precisely because coitus itself has something that is offensive for a woman. Both men and women struggle to avoid a passive position, as Freud himself remarked later in his life. But whereas the man can escape it due to the male anatomical function, a woman cannot, and so having sex with a man is always somehow difficult and 'dangerous'. For the woman, heterosexuality has the flavour of submission, something that the human being tends to resist. As we can see, we can find something 'unnatural', a struggle to adapt, even in what seems to be the most natural thing in the world: a woman lending herself to sexual intercourse.

This is why much of contemporary feminism has, in effect, glorified lesbian love, implying that a woman's sexual relations with men may be tolerated, but she herself cannot take pride in this. Hence, the feminist celebration of the clitoris, precisely because it does not serve as a complement to the male.[25] More broadly, male-female complementarity is essentially a moral ideal in our societies, not an inherent truth or a natural starting point.

Perversions, a Male Thing

In fact, Freud went on to distinguish between three types of masochism: erotic, feminine, and moral.[26]

Erotic masochism is the masochism of the perversion that goes by that name, of the kind that men usually enact with specialised prostitutes; we could simply call it *male masochism.* We have already discussed *female masochism.* Is it what makes all females desire a masochistic one? It is interesting, however, that Freud cites the case of a man as an example of female masochism. Evidently, female masochism is a problem only when a man expresses it, whereas for a woman it is deemed 'normal'.

As for *moral masochism*, Freud could find no erotic benefit in it, no utilitarian aspect. It is the tendency of some people, both men and women, to make sure that everything goes wrong in their lives, even to destroy themselves. Not to punish themselves, but … Freud can only invoke something un-analysable. He explains this dark desire for failure and self-destruction with the *death drive,* that is, he fails to explain it. The death drive is everything that is non-analysable. For this reason, whenever an analyst says of an analysand who is a source of great trouble, such as through a negative therapeutic reaction, that the death drive is acting upon them, what they are effectively saying is 'psychoanalysis is incapable of treating this person'. *Death drive* means the intrinsic limit of any psychoanalytic performativity.

With regard to female masochism, Freud's pupil Helene Deutsch,[27] more royalist than the king, went so far as to say that female pleasure is based entirely on masochistic fantasies: women imagine being raped, or being a prostitute, or in labour pains. However embarrassing these theses are for most women, they give substance to Freud's insinuation that masochism is something constitutive of femininity. Anyway, the question remains: if woman is 'normally' masochistic, why does she not engage in other perversions?

One could argue that if the sexual fetish is an *ersatz* female penis, a woman does not need to be a fetishist since her partner already has a penis. The woman does not require the copy because she already has the original. But what about the sadistic woman or the *voyeuse* or the female paedophile?

We could take the idea of fetishism as a phallic substitute very far. Isn't the 'normal' attraction a man feels for a woman, when stripped down to the essence of what is *truly* attractive in a woman, the attraction for what the woman lacks – the penis? This is reminiscent of the syndrome of *negative fetishism*.

Krafft-Ebing spoke of 'negative fetish': this is when a man is aroused not by a part of a woman's body, but by a part that she lacks. For him to find a woman desirable, she must lack something.[28] For example, one male could only have sex with women if they lacked a leg or limped conspicuously; another was only aroused by cross-eyed women. Another perverse analysand said, 'What arouses me is a certain *sagging* in a woman' – by which he meant a lack of freshness, wrinkles, drooping breasts, signs of ageing. Faced with the beautiful young woman he became engaged to, his sexual desire for her quickly faded.

This fetishism of lack is the 'objectual' facet of the syndrome in which certain individuals can only live well if they lose a member. They manage to have something amputated – usually a limb – because only this bodily absence provides them with balance. For them, it feels as though by being amputated, they have finally settled a debt. This is not an erotic preference; this is the way these subjects can *consist* in themselves.

Does this then mean that we can see the 'normally straight' man as a kind of negative fetishist, who absolutely wants to give the woman what she lacks? In fetishism proper, the man wants to offer the woman compensation *before* coitus, whereas in what is called normal attraction the man wants to offer it *through the coitus.* Is normal male heterosexuality a specific form of fetishism selected by society or the species, or both, to ensure that ends meet – in other words, to ensure the reproduction of the human beings?

Nevertheless, the prevalence of perversions in men pushes us to conclude that perversions are a typical man's way of handling femininity, including the femininity in himself. We have said that the ultimate referent of every perversion is always, in some way, the woman. But if at the bottom woman is masochistic, as Freud believes, the real nagging concern of the pervert is: 'What must I do with a woman?'

Perversions exist among gay men too. For instance, from the famous FBI Behavioral Science Unit's research, we know that if a serial killer targets only young men, he very probably has a same-sex orientation.[29] In contrast, a heterosexual serial killer will typically target girls and young women. In this sense, perversion for a long time was considered a specifically male way of relating sexually to women only because the majority of perverts are rather oriented toward women. However, paraphilia reveals a distinctly unique relationship between the human male and his sexual partner – the person he desires sexually and could even love.

Stoller: Sex and Gender

Robert J. Stoller has shown how perversions are a way of expressing – but also of controlling and softening – a profound hostility towards the other. This hatred, evident in sadistic acts, permeates every form of perversion, which is always the result of an interaction between hostility and sexual desire. The pervert's partner, a woman – accomplice or victim – is a replacement for the parent, against whom paraphilic individuals manifest their resentment.

The angry hostility at play in perversions depends on the fact that at least one of the reference adults decided to deny a child's *gender identity* – as a matter of fact, masculinity. In short, mum and dad didn't like having a boy.

In fact, perverts often say that a parent, usually their mother, combed or dressed them up as girls when they were children.[30] And if a mother did not already have a daughter as well, she would express the ardent desire to have one.

But what are masculinity and femininity? Now, it's not enough to have a penis to be a man or a vagina to be a woman. All sexual deviance proves that more is needed for a subject with a particular *sex* to be accepted as a member of a particular *gender*. This is the founding gamble of psychoanalysis, which was born as a queer theory.

It is precisely on this crucial point that psychoanalysis as a whole agonisingly hesitates. One of Freud's dogmas is the fundamentally bisexual constitution of every human being. Being a 'normal' woman or man means that one of the two parts, male or female, prevails over the other. The other gender is not usually abolished, but, as in a bricolage, it merges into the predominant sexual identification. The psychoanalytical theory of both neuroses and perversions hinges on a dialectic between masculine and feminine. For example, hysterics are subjects who have great trouble accepting their 'feminine dominancy'.

The problem, however, is that Freud never really clarified what masculine and feminine meant for him – it is not clear, therefore, what this bisexuality is made up of. For psychoanalysis, sexual desire (libido) is not specifically masculine or feminine: sexual drives have no sex. What seems to count here about the difference between masculine and feminine is not the difference between convex and concave, but rather the role taken in an activity.

In biology today, masculine and feminine are identified by the type of gametes, sexual cells, that one has. Among frogs, neither sex possesses a penis. An individual with a high number of small gametes is called male, and an individual with a limited number of large gametes is called female.

Freud, instead, *in a certain sense* says that we can identify the masculine with activity and the feminine with passivity.[31] He thought that every drive has both an active and passive form: sucking and being sucked, defecating and receiving the excrement of others, looking and being looked at, attacking and being attacked, and so on. By 'femininity' could we then mean the passive version of the drive?

But Freud also says that every drive, as such, is in a certain sense active; it is a *doing*. The German *Trieb*, drive, is a masculine word. Every drive would therefore be masculine, including sexuality in women. The passive version of the drive should be: being sucked, being defecated on, being looked at, being penetrated, being attacked, and so on. Man gives and takes, while woman gives herself and lets herself be taken. Femininity is thus for Freud a specialisation of the masculine: *having something done to you.*

Freud's project was somewhat daring. On the one hand, he wanted to create psychoanalysis as a science; he wanted, in other words, to advance *universally valid* explanations of all human beings, past, present, and future. Yet his gamble was at the same time to historicise what we call identity – and in particular gender identity. In short, one is not born male or female; one becomes it. Psychoanalysis aims at the history of each individual – hence the analytical theories of libido evolution, of relation to castration, of the Oedipus complex and its destruction, and so on. These theories aim to show how a being with a certain type of body will psychically become a man or a woman – or something else – via a historical process marked by struggles, disappointments, and traumas.

In this history, anatomy does indeed play an essential role, but mainly as an experience of objective confrontation with the other's anatomy: it is essential, at a certain point, for the boy to discover that girls have no 'willy' and for the girl to discover that boys have something she does not. Freud wrote that 'anatomy is destiny', but in fact anatomy is just one of the variables.

This project is in obvious contradiction with the common sense of most biologists. It is difficult for a biologist to accept the idea that what differentiates males and females is only an anatomical difference, and that everything else is a history of desire. Hormonal differences also play a decisive role.

Anyway, the fact remains that the results of today's sophisticated tests, despite being equal for many registers – intelligence levels, for example – differ greatly between women and men in several abilities. Is it possible to explain this difference in terms of different paths of psychic formation? We have two contrasting points of view on this. Some scholars tend to radically historicise gender identity – like queer theorists – while others tend instead to universalise and naturalise the differences between males and females. For the latter, the historical and cultural variations we are able to document, however spectacular, are ultimately of little relevance.

Now, Freudian theory never really makes up its mind between the two approaches, the historicist and the naturalist. On the one hand, it aims at enunciating what is universal in humankind, and therefore refers everything back to the constitution – what today we call genetics – of *Homo sapiens*. On the other hand, it reconstructs the formation of gender belonging as an individual historical process. The original psychoanalytical theory oscillates between historical and genetic elements. For example, the development in Freud of the various libidinal phases – oral, anal, phallic – seems to depend on a genetic inscription. Thus, is the Oedipus complex inscribed in the psycho-biological destiny of every human being, or is it the milestone of an individual history? And if it is a product of individual history, how could it then occur universally and necessarily?

Stoller: Primary Femininity

Stoller addresses the rather overwhelming issue concerning the relation between sexuality and individual history.

As an answer to the enigma of bisexuality, he hypothesises, in contrast to Freud, a *primary* femininity, that is, as he defines it himself, a 'nuclear gender identity'. This identity does not depend on individual historical vicissitudes, but is inborn.

According to Stoller, however, femininity is primary: initially, we are all female. Then some of us acquire masculinity, usually individuals with a penis, but there are interesting exceptions, like transgenders. In Stoller's psycho-embryology, femininity is what we all inherit, and masculinity is something only some of us acquire. We are all born female, but some can become male. Therefore, Stoller thinks that some are females because they *remain* females: femininity is a failed development. And, indeed, to become men we need substantial help from our mothers.

We are all originally females because the first person we're in relation to is a woman: in the symbiotic, fusional relationship established between baby and mother, the former adopts the latter's femininity as a primary identity. Our first sex is our mother's.

But at this point Stoller becomes tangled up in his own strings. This primary femininity is apparently acquired in the relationship with the mother, but then he speaks of a biological masculinity too. This nuclear identity is supposedly to be seen in all the precocious differences in aptitude between males and females, differences that do not, therefore, derive from external influences. For example, newborn baby boys are more able than girls to raise their heads from the lying position; at 13 months, girls are more reluctant than boys to separate from their mothers; boys tend to fling their toys, girls to gather them together; and so on.

Now, these and other examples concern acts or tendencies *more or less* present in males and females, but that do not differentiate them category-wise. Is a lower or greater tendency to do something enough to determine a gender difference? And when in adulthood most men are attracted only to women and most women only to men, is this sharp division based on more or less marked tendencies?

Though he asserts the presence of a primary sexual identity, for Stoller what really counts remains *the mental history of an individual*, through which, though born a male, he can become an effeminate homosexual, or cross-dresser, or transperson. And for there to be a history – and hence the abandonment or betrayal of primary gender identity – there must be an intervention by the Alter. This Alter, in mainstream psychoanalysis, is the mother. If the individual abandons what she or he originally was, it is because the mother has *distorted* something primal.

As for the primitive relationship of the subject with the Alter, certain strands of psychoanalysis begin with an equally mythical assumption: *primal symbiosis with the mother*. The theory of symbiosis – according to which the infant's Self is initially not differentiated from that of the mother – was developed by some analysts (for example, by Margaret Mahler and Jane G. Goldberg) to replace another no less mythical assumption by Freud: that of *primary narcissism*, that is, of an infant originally preoccupied only with her or his body and needs. According to many analysts, the substantial progress psychoanalytic knowledge has made regarding small children has consisted in understanding that we were not originally closed into ourselves, but merged with the mother, and hence that maturing does not mean so much gradually *opening up to* others (as Freud thought) but rather *separating and distinguishing oneself from* the mother.

Now, this mythical primary symbiosis is invoked by Stoller to explain masculine homosexuality and transsexualism, which was called transgenderism later. In the symbiotic phase, the infant thinks *he or she is the mother*: the infant feels they are a part of the mother, and the mother is a part of them. And, because the mother is a female, the subject feels it is female. This would be a primal femininity, considered not as something that is in opposition to masculinity, but as an unlimited or indefinite something from which both femininity and masculinity derive. Therefore, the fact that later in life a male feels feminine is a relic of this primal femininity based on maternal imprinting. But this theory encounters serious difficulties.

First of all, the fact that the mother is a woman does not *ipso facto* imply that maternal functions are feminine. Feminine functions and motherly functions do not coincide. If, like Freud, we think of masculinity as activity, we should qualify maternal functions as masculine: who is more active than a mother, who is more passive than a newborn? The mother–infant relation appears as a complementary relationship where the mother plays the active role. If the infant identified with the mother, he would identify with eminently active functions. Unless Stoller means that the infant identifies – or psychologically fuses – not with the mother as a mother, but with the mother as a woman. In this case, we would adopt an entirely different perspective, because the infant would then be able to see the mother as a woman too, that is, as someone outside their relationship.

After all, an adult who does not emerge from the symbiotic stage, who cannot differentiate him or herself as an autonomous Self, would be a thoroughly backward individual or a schizophrenic, while effeminate men and transpersons are, of course, usually by no means backward or schizophrenic. How to deal, then, with the theory of primary symbiosis?

Greenacre comes to our aid with her theory of *focal symbiosis*: the effeminate homosexual's or the transsexual's mother is unable to solve a symbiosis focused on sexual traits.[32] But why continue to use the term symbiosis, which always implies something total and pervasive and by no means something focal? A focal symbiosis is an oxymoron. Stoller's theory remains full of holes.

Judith Butler and Gender Hegemony

The fundamental distinction advanced by Stoller between sex and gender went on to gain remarkable prominence in the decades that followed, especially in the Anglo-American context, to the point that the category of sex is almost sidelined by that of gender. When a child is born, people no longer ask, 'What sex is it?' but rather, 'What gender should be assigned?' And there is an increasing tendency to distinguish sex from sexuality. The latter is taken to be sexual drives and, more broadly, everything related to the erotic body. Sex, by contrast, is taken to imply a binary division that is seen, in some ways, as arbitrary – a matter of assignment, that is, an imposition of signifiers onto human beings who are, at their origin, queer.

If *gender* is understood as something historically constructed, on the other hand, it loses almost all connection with *sexuality*. This completely overturns Freud's claim that 'anatomy is destiny'.

One of the most influential figures in advancing the concept of *gender* is Judith Butler.[33] A feminist activist, Butler was deeply influenced by psychoanalysis, particularly Lacan's, and more broadly by French post-structuralism. I said that Freud's own theory of sexuality is fundamentally queer. For Freud, sexual drives have no inherent sex; they are neither masculine nor feminine. Human beings are, at their core, 'polymorphously perverse'. For Freud too, identification with genders is a construction, though not in the sense implied by gender theory: it is a process that takes shape across the course of individual history, through a subjective encounter between one's own body and the bodies of others. What Freud does not consider are the various cultural contexts in which femininity and masculinity are conceived. Butler, by contrast – along with other radical gender theorists – emphasises the *social* construction of *gender*.

Butler articulates a way of thinking that goes well beyond philosophy and psychoanalysis, and today permeates much of contemporary thought about the world: social constructivism. That is, any so-called 'natural' difference between human beings – especially that of gender – is rather a social product, the result of the cultural pressures to which we are subjected. The constructivist claims: 'the culture we grow up in is our destiny'. All the psychic and emotional traits we attribute to the 'feminine' and the 'masculine' are not the product of natural sexual differences (anatomical or hormonal) but of the *performative* power of social identifications. At bottom, this view holds to the *omnipotence* of the social over individuals: everything we are derives not from our genes or from our bodies, but from the paradigms of different cultures.

Butler takes up the concept of the *performative* from John Austin, one of the founders of analytic philosophy. He drew attention to the *practical*, and thus concrete, dimension of language: *we can do things with words.*[34] If I say to someone, 'In a few days I will kill you', I am not merely informing him that I intend to kill him; rather, I am enacting a *threat*, which is a kind of promise. This speech act identifies me as *the one who threatens* and the other as *the one who is threatened*; something that is not without consequences.

We can argue that almost all our speech is performative; social life is woven from such acts. In short, the Alter almost always addresses me performatively, so I am constructed by the word of the Alter. And often it will be a matter of deconstructing what I have become through the Alter's identifying word. Gender theory focuses on gender performativity.

If we say to a female child, 'you're a little girl, and you will become a woman', she will indeed end up feeling herself to be a woman. She will be convinced that she will desire men, she will scream in fear if she sees a spider, she will prefer to study psychoanalysis rather than engineering, and so on, because she feels herself to be *naturally* a woman. As we can see, Butler's constructivism takes seriously the fundamental difference between *nature* and *nurture*, between biological reality and cultural processes, making the second term of the distinction clearly prevail over the first. Natural differences are almost irrelevant; what counts is what social violence will turn us into.

With a sophisticated vocabulary borrowed from the philosophy of language, Butler underscores the near-omnipotence of cultural performativity in shaping our identity – an idea characteristic of 20th-century culture. In psychology, for example, attachment theory is highly influential today: it holds that the essential is decided by the way a mother and her young child interact. 'We are the product of our mum' is a more family-centred version of the same constructivist view that 'we are all products of social performativity'.

In opposition to this tendency, another approach stresses above all the genetic inheritance of each of us.[35] According to this view, processes of socialisation are themselves conditioned by 'nature', which today means our genome. From this perspective, it is mistaken to think that schizophrenia or autism results from the mother–child relationship or from social performativity; rather, they are both effects of the individual's genome. Hence, the many studies cited on identical twins, who tend to manifest the same disorders even when they have lived apart since early childhood (quite a rare sample, in fact). To this, social constructivists reply with the many cases of identical twins who grew up together yet ended up leading entirely different lives. The debate continues.

I personally reject both theses, since they take the categorical distinction between nature and culture too literally. One current lets nature prevail, another culture. But matters are far more complex. We must find a way out of the trap of this dichotomy.

There is an evident anthropological fact: the modes of being feminine, like the modes of being masculine, change – sometimes quite dramatically – across different epochs and societies. What is there in common between an Afghan woman who accepts wearing a burqa and submitting to the power of bearded men, and a modern feminist woman in a major industrial metropolis who is a university dean? The question to which social constructivism offers no answer is: what has made it the case that in certain societies one model prevails, while in others a very different one takes root?

Every culture includes exceptions, of course. Today, trans people stand at the centre of philosophical admiration, for their existence shows the impossibility of reducing sexuality to the gender binary. Yet every epoch and society has had its trans people. Native Americans, for instance, recognised the *Two-spirit* men – referred to as *berdaches* by the French – who dressed as and lived as women.

Not all cultures follow a patriarchal model. Some societies are in a certain sense matriarchal – assuming that the concept of *matriarchy* can be applied to societies whose categories differ greatly from our own. The Nah or Mosuo, a people of some tens of thousands living in China, are often cited in this regard. In their peaceable society, a form of *gynocracy* prevails where power is exercised by women. The argument goes: if *one* human society functions through the political primacy of women, then in principle any society could function in the same way.

In sum, whether we are dealing with individual or cultural variations, human freedom is immense – though not that of individuals, but that of societies. Individual 'spirits' have little freedom to manoeuvre, whereas the Objective Spirit, as Hegel called it, has absolute freedom. The Objective Spirit is everything that constitutes our institutions and social rules. Yet the great freedom that a culture (Objective Spirit) possesses results in an overwhelming cultural domination over individuals.

The mere fact that gynocratic societies, or societies absolutely egalitarian in terms of gender (as ours is gradually becoming), are possible does not mean that they are *the most probable*. In short, the freedom to construct different social models – and therefore different sexualities – is constrained by factors that determine the greater or lesser *probability* of certain configurations.

For example, some societies – such as the Trobriand Islanders studied by Bronisław Malinowski – do not recognise symbolic kinship between fathers and children: the father is considered merely the mother's husband. There are also societies that do not recognise mother–child kinship, that is, mothers are considered wombs for rent, as some might put it today; apparently, this was the case in ancient Sparta. But it would be mistaken to conclude that cultures therefore have unlimited freedom in defining kinship, completely ignoring the physical processes of conception and generation. Such cases, where biological functions are symbolically inverted, are rare. In general, cultural differences – in kinship as in gender – take into account the probabilities that certain psychological traits correspond to a given anatomy.

Culture does tend to draw sharp lines where in nature there is a continuous process. For example, in our societies, legal adulthood begins at 18: on that very day, a citizen acquires certain fundamental adult rights. In reality, of course, the maturation process is much less sharply defined; it is a continuous development – or may not occur at all in certain individuals. Yet this does not mean that everyone, from a 10-year-old girl to a 50-year-old woman, should be regarded as adults alike. Today, we think that at 18 there is a higher probability that a citizen has reached adulthood in the sense we understand it. In other words, culture does not impose absolutely arbitrary distinctions.

In sum, culture structures natural variations – including sexual differences – in very different ways. But the great variety of 'readings' of continuous processes through discontinuous signifiers is never entirely free. Every culture interprets nature, so that in the end we can no longer tell to what extent certain differences are due to nature or to culture; that is, in the final outcome it is practically impossible to separate what results from social pressure from what derives from natural dispositions. We cannot ignore certain original dispositions, even if they may be culturally reinforced or tempered. Natural differences, including hormonal ones, often assert themselves *in resistance* to cultural prescriptions. Human beings are not *blank slates* in relation to performative acts.

For example, the anthropologist Emmanuel Todd cites what he was told by the head of a team of prehistoric anthropologists.[36] This team set itself the task of reproducing the most primitive artefacts – spears and pots – using the same materials and techniques of that time. Archaeological evidence indicates that men specialised in working stones to make spear and arrow points, while women specialised in shaping pots. The team leader observed that male researchers likewise preferred to fashion spear points, while female researchers gravitated toward pottery. That these forms readily evoke the essential shapes of male and female genitalia adds, perhaps, a 'Freudian' dimension to this difference in preferences. It is important to stress that these are *preferences*, not a form of determinism.

Overall, there appears to be a female tendency toward concave forms and a male tendency toward convex ones. And this difference requires explanation. It cannot be reduced simply to the effect of performative education. Even if it were, we would still need to understand why this educational pressure works for some individuals, but little or not at all for others.

Every human culture is, in a sense, an experimental variation. That is, humans have not discovered an optimal form of social life, nor an optimal way of recognising genders, toward which all societies naturally gravitate. Since every society must rely on some form of division of labour to function, they tend to assign different tasks to the genders in a fairly clear-cut way – just as we divide the continuum of individual maturation at the age of 18. In so-called 'primitive' societies, men mostly hunted while women gathered and devoted themselves to endless cooking. There were undoubtedly some women who preferred hunting and some men who preferred gathering, but the prescription of gendered divisions of labour was not purely arbitrary. It must be said, however, that culture often reinforces what are initially rather small differences. Thus, there are societies in which men engage almost exclusively in hunting and warfare, while women are permitted only to gather, care for children, and cook. These extreme societies, however, are not the product of some mysterious oppressor of women (and men) who descended from the sky. (Even today, the country with the highest proportion of female hunters registered with hunting associations is the United States: according to the 2024 US Fish & Wildlife Report, women account for 17% of all members. This is by no means a negligible minority, but it remains a minority nonetheless.)

In conclusion, philosophers such as Butler are not primarily concerned with understanding the origins of the variations in gender assignments across different epochs and cultures. Their focus is instead on a militant political strategy. They argue that it is necessary to show that other ways of living sexuality are possible, and on this point I agree. But the theory on which this militancy rests, namely the preponderance of culture over every aspect of human life, is flawed.

Notes

1 American Psychiatric Association (2022).
2 World Health Organization (2018).
3 Money (1988, p. 214).
4 Deleuze (1971).
5 Krafft-Ebing (1893); Ellis (1897); Moll (1893); Hirschfeld (1910, 1914); Binet (1887, 1888).
6 See G. Lanteri-Laura (1979).
7 Ballard (1973). This novel was later adapted into a film of the same name by David Cronenberg in 1996.

8 Lykins and Cantor (2013).
9 Mills (1993).
10 I will use the term 'modernised societies' to refer to those with the highest GDP per capita, governed by liberal pluralist democracies.
11 Karras (2005, p. 113).
12 Bentham (1789, p. 1).
13 Freud (1905d).
14 Wordsworth (1807), 'My Heart Leaps Up'.
15 Deleuze and Guattari (1972).
16 Deleuze and Guattari (1972, p. 231).
17 Freud (1927e).
18 Riviere (1929).
19 Benvenuto (2016).
20 Freud (1924c).
21 Especially in *Beyond the Pleasure Principle* (Freud, 1920g).
22 Freud (1920a) analysed the case of a young lesbian.
23 Réage (1967).
24 Current research (Critelli and Bivona, 2008) indicates that between 31% and 57% of women have fantasies in which they are forced into sex against their will, and for 9% to 17% of women these are a frequent or favourite fantasy experience.
25 See Malabou (2022).
26 Freud (1924c).
27 Deutsch (1944, 1945).
28 Krafft-Ebing (1893).
29 Ressler, Burgess, and Douglas (1988).
30 Stekel (1930); Stoller (1968, 1975).
31 Freud (1905d, 1915c).
32 Greenacre (1959).
33 Butler (1990).
34 The title of his seminal work on speech acts is 'How to Do Things with Words' (Austin, 1962).
35 A very well-known populariser of this perspective is Steven Pinker (2003).
36 Todd (2023).

Chapter 2

The Sadist's (In)Justice

The Apathetic Sadist Passion

By sadistic behaviour, we mean the enjoyment derived from inflicting suffering on another person. However, we have distinguished between a non-perverse form of sadism and one that is indeed perverse—just as Freud distinguished three types of masochism, although only one, erotic masochism, is properly a perversion. Non-perverse sadism can be described as an *enjoyment derived from cruelty*, fuelled by hatred and anger towards someone. What we will focus on here, instead, is erotic sadism, which aims to torment *a woman* precisely because she is attractive – or an attractive man, in the case of male sadistic homosexuals. In this instance, the sadistic act quite explicitly substitutes the amorous act.

We will not dwell on the psychoanalytic schools that view sadism and masochism not *per se*, but as correlated with other aspects of the personality that these schools consider more important than the Freudian libidinal dynamic. A well-established trend in psychoanalysis, for instance, places the greatest emphasis on the *narcissistic structure* of the subject, although narcissism is conceptualised differently across various schools (Self Psychology, Object Relations, and others). For Otto Kernberg,[1] in particular, sadism is inherent in the psychodynamics of what he calls *malignant narcissism*, which is the bridge connecting antisocial and narcissistic character dimensions. The malignant narcissist's antisocial behaviour is inflamed by ego-syntonic aggression and sadism.[2] Other trends view sadistic acts from the

DOI: 10.4324/9781003531388-2

perspective of developmental psychology or as an aspect of borderline personality.[3] But not all psychoanalytic schools (Lacanian ones among others) accept the borderline as a useful diagnostic concept.

Although these schools have made important contributions to the understanding of perversions, we will not discuss them here, as they do not assign particular significance to sexuality in the broader sense; in other words, they do not consider the specifically male nature of perversions. In this respect, they are removed from the original Freudian inspiration. From the outset, our approach has instead focused on *sexual* perversions, and therefore on sadism as an effect of the problematic relationship men have with women and with their sexual partner more generally.

In the Quentin Tarantino film *Death Proof* (2007), we find a rather unpleasant-looking stuntman with a scar on his face who has never had much luck with girls. Instead, he occasionally kills them in his modified car. It is a deliberately lowbrow slasher movie devoid of any psychological subtlety, yet it captures the way the common opinion interprets sadistic acts, primarily perpetrated against women: those who feel rejected by the female sex take out their frustration on surrogate women.

Hence the common premise: 'I, the sadist, find enjoyment in inflicting pain on a woman in order to punish Woman for her original "betrayal" – for enjoying another and not me'. Sadistic rape, in particular, would be an application of the law of retribution:

> My primal woman (my mother) will now pay for the pleasure she enjoyed with her man or another son, at the mercy of me (the excluded child), enduring a violent sexual act and the pain that the whore deserves for refusing to enjoy me when I was a child.

According to this view, the driving force of sadism is resentment.

Yet sexual sadism is a little more complicated. Sadism does not seem to be a form of revenge because the sadist actually feels no resentment towards his victim. This *apathy* on the part of the torturer – which we find throughout the works of the Marquis de Sade, from whom the term sadism is derived – is an essential characteristic of sadism. But in what way is the true sadist apathetic? Sadism is, in fact, a *pathos*, a passion; put simply, a way of deriving enjoyment. How can a *pathos* be apathetic?

Clavreul cites the testimony of a pair of sadistic murderers during their trial in the mid-1960s.[4] The peak of their pleasure did not come so much from the contemplation of their victim's suffering as from the *certainty of their innocence*. 'Much more than the victims' cries of pain', writes Clavreul, 'what matters to the sadist are the protestations of innocence and pleas for forgiveness'. That is to say, the sadist puts himself in the place of someone punishing a wrongdoer who must seek forgiveness. The humiliating helplessness of the other is far more enjoyable for the sadist than the other's physical suffering.

A sadistic act is not simply a muscular venting of rage. It is a *moral act*: innocence and guilt are concepts that imply a moral law, which is applied here ironically. In fact, the sadist stages a punishment ritual, albeit an inverted one. This recalls a passage from *The Adventures of Pinocchio*,[5] when the puppet ends up before a court in a strange land where the court immediately punishes those who declare their innocence. Consider, too, the inscription at the entrance to the Buchenwald extermination camp, *Jedem das Seine* ('To each his own'). For the Nazis, the Jews and other 'cursed' races or individuals deserved pain and extermination. The sadist, too, fundamentally experiences the sadistic act as a punishment that he must inflict … on the innocent. And so – like any executioner worthy of that name – he must not feel any personal animosity towards his victim. Alternatively, the sadist who 'takes *justice* into his own hands' derives enjoyment from the manifest *injustice* of which he is the agent. Here, he does not merely vent an original resentment; he presents himself as the hero of injustice, drawing upon himself all the resentment of those who suffer undeservedly. In this sense, the sadist operates in an almost philosophical scenario, one conceived by the Marquis de Sade (1740–1814): the sadist becomes an instrument, a secular arm, of the evil, metaphysical cruelty of Nature.

In an essay on Sade, Pierre Klossowski saw in the Sadean world a *male cruelty against the mother*. In this view, sadism lays bare not so much the Oedipus complex as a configuration we might call the Orestes complex, in which the hero kills the shameless mother, Clytemnestra, to vindicate the father. While it is true that the victims of Sade's heroes are both male and female, all of them nonetheless have a feminine quality. Women are the quintessential victims of the sadist. Except in the case of homosexual sadists.[6]

The old joke about a sadist and a masochist meeting, where the masochist says 'Hurt me' and the sadist joyously replies 'Never!', makes little sense unless the sex of the two characters is specified. The masochist must be a man and the sadist a woman. But the task of the sadistic dominatrix is not so much to inflict pain but rather to humiliate and frustrate her client, denying him intercourse. A dominatrix who, like the one in the joke, refuses to inflict pain on the masochist would likely be in great demand.

The Sadean torturer displays all the traits of an anarchic, lawless, arbitrary father who allies himself with filial female figures – the knavish Juliette of some of Sade's novels, for example – to torture a mother and subject her to all kinds of abuse. This anti-maternal constellation can also shed light on the petty sadism so often reported in the media, particularly in the case of sexual serial killers.

One of the most infamous sadists of all time is Jack the Ripper. At the time, in London's seedy Whitechapel district, five to seven prostitutes were murdered and their bodies horribly mutilated. The expert manner in which the victims were cut up suggested that the killer was either a butcher or a surgeon. The Ripper was never found.[7]

Were the victims all prostitutes simply because they were the most exposed and defenceless targets? Yet a comparison with similar cases suggests that massacres committed with the meticulousness of a ritual hinge on the relationship between sexuality and morality. Was the choice of prostitutes as victims merely practical? In fact, a punitive, purifying passion transpires from these murderous acts. Behind these rigorous executions lurks the misogynistic shadow of Raskolnikov, the hero of Dostoyevsky's *Crime and Punishment*,[8] who kills an elderly loan shark and her sister, who happens to be at the scene of the crime, as a form of moral protest against human evil. Especially female evil, it should be noted.

The exclusion of any experienced resentment, *distantiation*, is central in both masochism and sadism. The masochist usually feels no bitterness towards the woman who must abuse him, and the sadist is calm and serene before his victim. Yet psychoanalysis suggests that this very resentment, which is never perceived, is the driving force behind the sadomasochistic machine: *the act* replaces any *feelings* of anger or resentment. The original affects are replaced by the enjoyment associated with the act. And this is true of all perversions: they abolish the affect (passivity) in favour of activity. Anger, vexation, and resentment are in fact still affects, afflictions. Perversion is a paradoxical passion: it excludes passivity; it is always an *acting*. Masochists too, the apparent champions of passivity, are supremely active: the decision to be flogged and humiliated is theirs, it is they who call the shots by turning the gun on themselves.

Lacan and Sade's Fantasy

Lacan developed an original theory of sadomasochism (SM) based on the figure of the Marquis de Sade.[9]

Lacan says that we need to distinguish between the heroes of Sade's novels – who act out a hyperbolically sadistic desire – and the Marquis himself, whose existence actually makes him a champion of masochism. Sade was thrown into prison for some rather tame libertine games. The point is that he then did his best to remain confined for most of his life – mostly in the Bastille, and for 12 years in the lunatic asylum at Charenton.

In the wake of the psychoanalytic tradition, Lacan believes that sadism and masochism are correlated, i.e. that the sadist is also a masochist and vice versa. The sadist and the masochist change roles. Sadism and masochism are then the same acts seen from

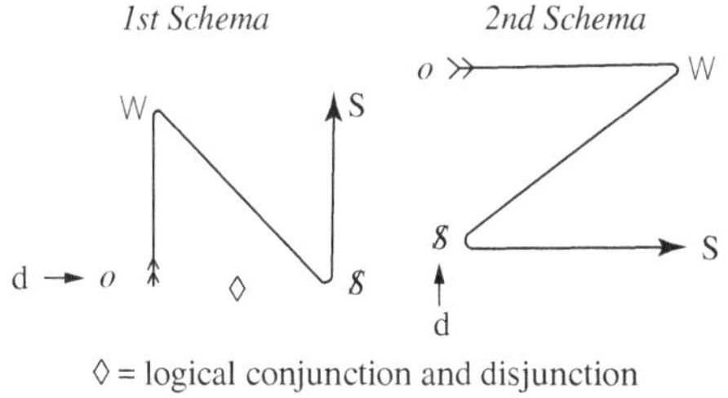

Figure 2.1 The Sadean-Fantasy Schema

two different points of view. Besides, in Sade, sooner or later almost all sadistic perpetrators fall victim to other sadists.

According to Lacan, Sade inverts Kant.[10] The Kantian universal law, indifferent to the interests of individual subjects, is for Sade none other than Lady Nature, a feminine word in French. For the Divine Marquis (as he is called by many), Nature is identified with the *obligation to enjoy*. First, in the sense of the enjoyment of Nature in the subjective genitive sense, it is Nature that enjoys. It needs to destroy the living, preferably human beings, in order to recreate living beings. But also, in the sense that Nature obliges us to enjoy at the cost of the destruction of the other. Sadistic pleasure is like Kant's categorical imperative: it does not aim at the well-being of subjects, nor does it seek to preserve their lives, but it compels everyone to unconditionally become an object of pleasure for the other. The sadist, therefore, is the executor of the ruthless law of Madam Nature.

In every perversion, we must distinguish the character of the drama from its author or director: while Sade's drama is clearly sadistic, its director is masochistic.

The SM 'game' begins with *the other as object*: the sadist torturing his victims. It is the representation of this sadistic act that makes us appreciate, for example, the cruel scenes of a film: if we experience enjoyment that we classify as aesthetic, it is because something in our sense of horror elicits that enjoyment, even if it pushes the limits of what we can bear.

So many violent films or narratives claim to be exposés of moral teachings, yet they work precisely because they tap into our SM enjoyment. These staged atrocities effectively split us in two. One side of us experiences the horrifying scenes as if we were witnessing them in real life and recoils in rejection. Another side – the 'aesthetic' – values them as powerful and as having an impact on the viewer. One side of us rebels against the torment, while the other takes enjoyment in it. By delegating evil to a fictional villain, we allow ourselves to enjoy the sadistic act, all the while seeing ourselves as potential victims who, deep down, take comfort in not being the actual ones.

Ultimately, every tragic or horror drama stages SM scenes. Our desire for 'intense emotions' through audiovisual media reveals our veiled desire for SM acts.

Lacan describes the sadist agent as an object, and not, as one would expect, a subject, because for him the true subject ($\$$) is the victim. A subject is almost by definition subjected. Just as in the many crucifixion scenes found in art, the *subject* we identify with is Christ on the cross. This split that Lacan addresses clearly permeates the Christian drama of the torture on the cross. The tormentors are only an instrument for the Passion of Christ, mere agents/objects. Now, for Lacan, the subject, like Christ on the cross, is fundamentally split. In the case of Sade, this split occurs because, on the one hand, the subject is subjugated to the torturer, obeying the law that commands: 'Make yourself the object of the enjoyment of the Other, the torturer'. Sade's paradoxical law is that any person, no matter who, must become the object of the other's enjoyment, even at the cost of suffering the most terrible tortures. And yet, on the other hand, everything in the object rebels against suffering.

Prostitutes mention clients who ask to enact a rape. The sex worker has to pretend she is being forced into sexual intercourse by the client, and scream. But usually, the man also insists that the woman scream with pleasure during the simulated rape, that she experience an inappropriate enjoyment. In other words, the sadist imagines a woman who discovers she herself is a masochist, that is, from his perspective, the ultimate woman. It is a rather tame form of sadism, aimed at rousing the subject into a tremendous orgasm. The point is that both suffering and enjoyment split the subject: in both cases, the subjects come out of themselves and, somehow, come into contradiction with themselves. The scream, whether of horror or pleasure, excites those who, like the sadist, cannot bear the other subject *that is in themselves.* In the case of simulated rape, the division is between the role of the victim and the impudent orgasm, which contradicts the first role.

This simulation is different from actual rape, where the rapist, alone or in a group, does not seem to care in the least about the victim's affects. The victim appears to be a mere object of enjoyment. But a more subtle analysis of real rape would lead us to distinguish between different types of aggression. Group abuse seems to revolve around an almost ritual punishment of the woman. But what is the woman guilty of? Obviously of not submitting to Sade's law, which prescribes that everyone become the object of the other's enjoyment whenever and wherever the other wishes. Women, in contrast, enjoy the overwhelming power of choosing who can enjoy them and who cannot. Sexuality places each subject at the mercy of the other, who therefore has an extraordinary power. Unlike other pleasures, sexual enjoyment usually requires the consent and participation of the other.

Love relationships, outside of pure fusional idylls, are often a battleground for power: the other has the power to offer me pleasure and happiness, but I too hold this power over the one who desires and loves me. Which of us desires or loves the other *more*? If I realise that I am more important to the other than they are to me, I will be very tempted to exploit this imbalance and subject them to all kinds of emotional blackmail.

Against this backdrop of power struggle, the rape of women by men becomes an act of war against female power: sexual violence is here a political act. Because all sadism is authorised by a law which, however heinous – like the law dictated by Sade – legitimises the torture of the guilty other. For the rapist, the woman is guilty of innocence.

In other words, for Lacan the sadistic agent (*a*) does not act directly on the subject-victim; the abuse obeys a Will (W) that is somehow transcendent, the Will of Nature. In Sade, the victim's suffering at the Will of Nature, a ruthless mistress, takes on a utopian perspective. The victim is split because, on the one hand, they are reduced to pure suffering, an inarticulate cry in which they lose all dignity and humanity: hyperbolic suffering leads first to the death of the victim's subjectivity, then to their physical death. In sadistic action, therefore, there is a yearning to annihilate suffering itself: in perspective, as the end result of Sade's fantasy, we find a mythical subject of pure enjoyment.

Who then desires what in sadism? In Sade's work, the focus is on the executioner, who derives pleasure from causing the victim to suffer by creating a split in them. But the psychological interpretation is only one of many. Osama bin Laden certainly organised the destruction of the Twin Towers, not least because it gave him enjoyment. When we look back at the images of the devastation of 9/11 and find ourselves both horrified and fascinated, we can interpret the whole through a masochistic lens: we identify with the many victims trapped in that living hell. The plethora of Hollywood disaster movies that anticipated such scenarios tapped into both the audience's masochistic readiness to empathise with the victims and the unconfessed sadism that makes us take enjoyment in witnessing slaughter.

But we can also look at 9/11 in non-psychological terms; in terms of a transcendent Will (W) beyond Al Qaeda and its leaders: the supposed will of Allah himself, who demands jihad. For supporters of Islamic fundamentalism, far from being a sadistic scene, it is simply a glorious moment that will lead to the planetary triumph of a holy model of society. The sadistic and masochistic 'ecstasies' are mere moments of this super-fantasy.

The sadist is then an agent of the law, of both the just law and the evil law. In the latter, the innocence of the victim is their deepest source of enjoyment.

A subject in analysis would often tell me how he loathed children, especially boys. This jeopardised his marriage, since his wife wanted a child, while the mere idea sickened him. Once, he was walking with his wife and, upon seeing a child with his mother in the street, he suddenly blurted out that he wanted to kick the boy and crush his head until his brains splattered out. At first, I thought he was acting out his aggression towards his younger sister – he had reacted to her arrival quite badly when he was a child. But this presumed fixation on the trauma of his sister's birth clashed with the fact that the targets of his horrifying fantasies were primarily male children.

He said he hated children because he thought they were selfish and whimsical, demanding everything from their mothers here and now, unmindful of the needs of others, and 'strong with the weak and weak with the strong'. As he made his list of grievances, it became clear to me that, in a sense, the child he was describing was actually himself, as he still was as an adult. I realised that the hateful child he wanted to torture was a sort of mirror projection of himself, even though he didn't recognise it as such.

Is it then enough to say here that these sadistic fantasies referred to actual masochistic experiences? It is not in any reversal of roles that we find the essential dynamics of sadism. In fact, the patient was aware of the sadistic fantasies that he had been nurturing since childhood – also in relation to that party pooper of a little sister. His sadistic fantasies were sadism to the nth degree: they undertook to punish a selfish, mean, substantially sadistic, and by no means innocent child. In general, the innocence to torture sadistically is the reverse of guilt: sadists never cease to persecute their own sadism, taking enjoyment in doing so.

But ultimately, at the root of this guilt lies an almost metaphysical injustice, which Sade theorised in his own way, based on delirious philosophy: the cosmic injustice of a cruel stepmother, Nature. The sadist wants to somehow satiate the evil hunger of nature, even though he may fall victim to it himself. It would be no mistake to say that at the core of sadism lies a thirst for revenge against a hideous mother who has failed us – except that the sadist adapts to this maternal injustice, to its sovereign arbitrariness, by tormenting creatures innocent and guilty like himself.

Then, is presenting oneself as an avenger of justice – or injustice – merely the sadist's moral alibi? But why should the sadist, unlike so many other perverts, have this particular vocation to rationalise and exculpate himself? Exhibitionists or voyeurs, if caught, will not attempt to justify their actions. In short, the sadist is never *pure*: being instrumental to a law – even the unjust and cruel law of Lady Nature – is not an alibi for sadism but one of its constitutive elements. This is what Lacan denotes as the transcendent Will, of which the sadist becomes at once impersonator, executor, and instrument.

The Third Reich tried to build consensus around its policies of eliminating the mentally ill with a series of films. One of these films revolves around the following situation: a very likeable Aryan neurologist realises that a degenerative brain disease will soon cause his mind to deteriorate irreparably. He therefore asks his colleagues to do him the favour of eliminating him. (Note that for Nazi psychiatry, just as for today's dominant psychiatry, all mental illnesses are due to a broken brain.) Moral: by killing the mentally ill, the state is merely fulfilling the will of the ego. This ruthlessness is portrayed as an act of compassionate euthanasia. It would be naïve to dismiss this as 'mere propaganda designed to make an abhorrent policy morally acceptable'. Rather, it is likely that National Socialists genuinely thought along the lines of these films. Here, too, the extermination of the weak is carried out in the name of a sublime Will – that of the fair-haired, blue-eyed man in possession of his full mental faculties.

A Perverse Theory of Perversions?

In contrast to the dominant psychologism in psychoanalysis, Lacan undoubtedly brings to light the properly ethical dimension of perversions. In sum, the perverse are not animals who get up to all sorts of mischief without regard for laws and rules; on the contrary, they enjoy submitting to the law. The sadist does not break the law any more than a petty thief does in order to make a living. Indeed, we see perversion in sadism but not in theft – except in the case of kleptomania, where we can grasp a perverse enjoyment. From a non-psychological perspective, a torturer finds enjoyment because he interprets the law sadistically: to him, the law is the enjoyment of the Alter.

This thesis should not surprise us, given that the history of Western thought is full of theories of law that make this very argument: legal systems are actually a way of ensuring the satisfaction of a privileged few. The Greek sophists – Polus, Callicles, Thrasymachus – already questioned whether the laws of the City were an expression of the strong, through which they maintained their hold on power, or whether they were a contrivance of the weak precisely to protect themselves from the power of the strong.

But the point is that the law is not ethics. Today, in many languages ethics is distinct from morals, a distinction parallel to that between legitimacy and legality. Legality is the system of laws, while legitimacy is an order that transcends the legal system: it is an unwritten principle that in turn judges the laws and recognises whether or not they are legitimate. The concept of legitimacy – of a law that judges the laws – evokes the ethical dimension of laws.[11] Now, in Lacan's reconstruction, what sadomasochism lacks is precisely the ethical dimension. Lacan's perverse are moralists at heart, but it is precisely for this reason that they will face prosecution.

In this theory, the other is either the Alter or an object *a*. The other is either the law, language (the treasure of signifiers), or Sade's Will of Nature – in short, something that transcends every subject – or it is the small object *a* that arouses and seduces me. In both cases, the other as subject – the other in whom I presume subjectivity – does not appear on the scene. It either exists as an object (and is therefore not really other from me, or other with respect to me, given that someone is always an object-for-a-subject), or it does not exist because it is Alter from every self. Indeed, according to Lacan the Alter does not *exist*, and to believe that it does is a delusion. The fact that it may be a position, a place, or an agent does not imply its existence. Because if it did exist, it would be an 'itself' and no longer an Alter. For Lacan, the Alter exists in the same way that the horizon line 'exists': the moment we want to incorporate that line into our own horizon to describe it, it ceases to be the horizon line, since our horizon has now shifted beyond it. In short, the horizon always marks the limit of *my* perspective. Lacan's Alter is not the other of intersubjectivity; it is always the Alter-for-a-subject. The Alter is like the reverse side of a glove: if we turn it inside out, it is no longer the reverse side but the right side.

So, does the ethical dimension of life lead us to assume that the other exists? In any case, we can never enjoy the ultimate evidence of this existence. What we ourselves see as evidence are only the behaviours of the other. So, do we enter an ethical dimension to the extent that we consider the subject that manifests itself in these behaviours as existing? An existence that binds and commits us? In other words, is ethics a system of laws, or is it based on the recognition of the reality of the other?

Now, in sadomasochism, the other is only *legal*, but the way the perverse person uses this other is always illegitimate, even when not punishable by law. Insofar as sadomasochists subject themselves to the law (otherwise they would not be able to find enjoyment), they lack the ethical relationship to the other. And every law is legitimate for us – i.e. ethical – to the extent that it makes the other present to us as existing, and not the reverse of the glove, the right side of which is us. But the point is: do human beings exist who are truly capable of *caritas*? This Latin word simply meant *love*.

The Martyred Female Saint

In many cases, the victims of sadistic violence are escorts. Why them in particular? The sadists who prey on these women seem to harbour a deep hatred, especially for the most destitute sex workers. The sadistic act is fundamentally an act *against* women, and it becomes even more brutal against women who sell their bodies for money.

As in the case of Jack the Ripper, an unyielding moral light radiates from these sadistic acts, a desire for purification against 'lost women'.

In truth, sadistic crimes against women – which often are serial crimes and could go on forever – aim to make all women, or rather Woman herself, suffer to the brink of death. This is the Sadean-metaphysical aura of sadism.

A dark criminal plot unfolds in the crimes of the 'Monster of Florence', who, in the province of the Tuscan city, between 1968 and 1985 murdered eight couples, often mutilating the bodies. 'He' would murder young couples who had retreated in search of intimacy, often just as they were about to engage in sexual intercourse. In four of the eight attacks, he sheared off the pubis of the girl, and in two cases he also severed the left breast. He would typically kill the man first, then drag the woman out of the vehicle or tent and brutalise her: he would perform a physical separation of the male and female bodies, symbolically annulling their carnal union.[12] The excision of the pubis and breasts proclaimed the desexualisation of the woman. Did the killer act solely out of envy of young couples who appeared to be living an erotic and amorous idyll? Or was he driven by an exaggerated, punitive mission against the 'sins of the flesh' committed by the young?

Sadistic resentment singles out the prostitute as the most innocent of women. The sadist's pleasure comes not from punishing the guilty – the ravishing beauty who gazes down on you with contempt – but from punishing the guiltless. The sadist is the ironic avenger of injustice.

The sadist particularly deplores those 'wretched prostitutes' who are also poor, because they also arouse what Adela Cortina has called *aporophobia*, fear and disgust for poor people.[13] The most widespread form of xenophobia is really an abhorrence of the poor; it is actually aporophobia. An equation emerges: the poor, especially if they are foreign, stink. Aporophobia is an epiphany of political vomiting. In fact, we vomit not only when we want to expel something revolting from our stomach, but also when we see something repulsive before us. Our eyes 'eat' even what nauseates us; the mere sight of what sickens us is itself an invasion of our body; and we have to throw up what has found its way inside us through our eyes or nostrils. And what we despise most is poverty. I see bitter hatred in many when they stumble upon vagrants, beggars, ragged immigrants in the street: the visible presence of the destitute is an attack on their respectability. As if being in proximity to the poor or deprived also infected them with poverty and deprivation.

On the contrary, official morality idealises the poor. It is something many eminent religious philanthropists have stated: the poor have the halo of the divine. Mother Teresa of Calcutta said that she saw the reflection of the face of Christ in every poor person. So, our culture experiences a lacerating contradiction. Xenophobic vomit somehow produces something of the divine.

But in the case of sadistic serial killers, aporophobia seems to be only the precondition for a more sophisticated passion. The sadist knows that 'the poor whore', more than any other poor person, is sacred.

For centuries, our culture has felt a deep ambivalence, not only towards the poor but also towards prostitutes. In moments of anger toward a woman, the words that roll from our lips are 'damned whore'. In short, 'whore' is something that today inspires increasing horror. While aporophobia is hushed, hypocritically unacknowledged, the pornophobic insult (*porné* in Greek meant prostitute) is instead permitted, uncensored. It serves as a sufficient substitute for blasphemy. The term 'whore' deftly slips into the place of God's name, yet somehow absorbs its majesty. The prostitute, in short, is the ultimate social abomination, but for that very reason she inspires a kind of holy respect.

Christian culture, which has nurtured us, even when we claim to be atheists, has always sanctified the prostitute. Starting with Mary Magdalene, who is never described in the Gospels as a prostitute but as a woman whom Jesus delivered from being possessed by seven devils. Yet for many centuries Christians have absolutely wanted to believe that Jesus' foremost female disciple, the first human being to have seen him resuscitated, was a whore.

Countless are the prostitutes or licentious women who become nuns and saints in Christian edifying literature. From Hrotswitha of Gandersheim to John Ford (in *Stagecoach*), paeans to the harlot have lauded the woman whom bourgeois morality relegates to the lowest rung of respectability. This *pornophilia* is continued in secular and modern fiction, for example, in the prostitute of *Crime and Punishment*, who redeems Raskolnikov by following him on his deportation to atone for his crime.

This radical ambivalence towards the prostitute generates an emotional whirlwind on which sadistic passion thrives.

Therefore, to inflict suffering on the whore is to brutalise the sacred side of the woman. As we have discussed, sadistic enjoyment lies above all in knowing that the victim's suffering is unjust and that it makes her a martyr. The sadistic 'retribution' is unfathomable: it brutalises not just any woman, but the *holy* woman. For it is only through the unjust punishment of poverty and innocence that the sadist renews and revives the deep wound around which his lechery erupts: the torment of being a male rejected by women, then as now. He too, like the prostitute, is the vomit of society, but he turns himself into a demon who inflicts pain and humiliation on the 'sacred' woman.

Notes

1 Kernberg and Yeomans (2013).
2 Sofra (2020).
3 Sehgal (2018).
4 Clavreul (1967, p. 100).
5 The novel by Carlo Collodi (2000).
6 Klossowski (1967).
7 On Jack the Ripper's case, see Sugden (1995).
8 Dostoyevsky (1866).
9 Lacan (1989).
10 Kant (1788).
11 On the difference between legitimacy and legality in legal theory, see Solum (2010).
12 On the Monster of Florence, see Giuttari (2006).
13 Cortina (2017).

Chapter 3

The Masochist's Strategy

The Humiliating Woman

As we have seen, Freud distinguishes between three forms of masochism. Here we shall concentrate on erotic masochism, which belongs most strictly to the area of perversion.

The affinity between the enjoyment of the masochist and the elevation of the pious soul through mortification has often been emphasised. This is what makes the figure of Francis of Assisi so fascinating and at the same time unsettling. He embraced the life of a beggar, inflicting on himself all kinds of humiliations. What he called 'perfect joy' – a state of spiritual delight – was only achieved through suffering, especially through acts of mortification. Towards the end of his life, Francis himself declared that the greatest joy he could imagine would be to be expelled from the Franciscan order he had founded and led.[1] The ultimate humiliation: to be cast out from his own creation.

With Francis we have a form of masochism that Freud seems not to have considered: it is by no means erotic, but neither is it feminine or moral. I would call it *spiritual masochism*. Perhaps there is something spiritual in all forms of masochism, even the 'common' masochism of those who seek out a prostitute for a flogging. In fact, according to a Lacanian approach, as we will see, all forms of perversion have a 'spiritual' ironic hard core: 'The Lord's Will be done'.

I will start with what I would call *the elementary masochistic fantasy*: a man enjoys suffering on account of the woman he loves. This suffering is rooted in an original betrayal: '*She, the cruel one,*

DOI: 10.4324/9781003531388-3

prefers another to me'. Yet, strangely enough, the spectacle of the pain and humiliation she inflicts does not make him hate this unyielding woman. He does not denounce the suffering and humiliation he endures for the supposed enjoyment of the woman; on the contrary, he somehow glorifies it.

In masochism, the transformation of exclusion into enjoyment is spectacular. I, the masochist, do not demand that the woman love, desire, or respect me – on the contrary, I wish her to beat and humiliate me. She must make her contempt for me unmistakable. And I enjoy this contempt. Why?

The masochist sometimes responds in a spiritual register: 'Through humiliation and pain, I elevate myself'. Dominatrices who advertise their services to masochistic clients in the media also promise '*discipline*'. Strict discipline elevates the spirit, granting access to a higher form of enjoyment born of sacrifice and humiliation.

The masochist takes no pleasure in physical pain as such. For him, pain is no more or less unpleasant than it is for everyone else. Pain takes on value only within an erotic context – where it becomes the condition for a surplus enjoyment. Physical pain is pleasurable only insofar as it is inflicted *by a woman* and only insofar as *it signifies* punishment and humiliation – that is, when pain is part of a moral act.

Even when the masochist has to make do with the collaboration of prostitutes, deep down, he dreams of a woman who is *truly* enraged with him and wants to punish him. However, even if the masochist did succeed in finding a woman genuinely furious with him, that charitable complementarity, capable of cancelling out the perverse strategy, would still not be achieved. In fact, a woman authentically angry with the subject would derive no particular pleasure from her state; quite the opposite. The subjugated subject desires an '*uncompromising*' woman (Italian prostitutes specialised in masochists often advertise themselves using this term), but he does not wish to satisfy her supposed desires. We label someone a masochist when the other's feelings are not *an end* for him – meaning that his goal would be to actualise them – but *a means* of procuring enjoyment only for himself. When the masochist declares himself to be the 'slave' of his 'mistress', he does not take enjoyment in fulfilling the woman's desire to be a dominatrix; rather, he only enjoys his *feeling* of being her slave. In the notation we have proposed, the compliant, 'strict' woman is an *alia*, but the *Alter* who must ultimately enjoy is the woman (the mother) who constantly seems to repeat to the subject: 'I want enjoyment! But *you* cannot give me enjoyment!'

A woman told her man he had a smaller-than-average penis, while she genuinely enjoyed very large penises. So, he arranged threesomes with men known to have large penises; he watched his woman have intercourse with these more endowed men and particularly liked the fact that his woman constantly made suggestive remarks comparing her partner's 'little willy' to that of the new lover. There was, however, one crucial condition: that she always chose him in the end. The masochist takes great risks, always counting on ultimate victory. As Theodor Reik (1953) wrote: 'The masochist loses all battles … except the last one'. In the end, he triumphs on the match point, the final moment when it is all or nothing.

An adult masochist began to have masochistic fantasies as a child. He was captivated by scenes in which the hero of the film was flogged and wounded by his enemies, and in his reverie he would put himself in the position of the protagonist. The figure of the bare-chested hero certainly had clear sexual undertones for him, something that could have led to a homosexual outcome in adulthood, though this didn't turn out to be the case. What was important, however, was that the positive hero of the film, the one destined for the happy ending, was tortured, humiliated, or injured. Pain and humiliation, in short, are the path to perfect dominance and joy. The masochist is in most cases a grandiose man who needs to dominate by risking everything, as we see in most action films. Adventure films where the hero seems to be plunged into the depths of his own defeat appeal to many, but *being the hero* who risks it all is what attracts the masochist.

The masochistic *mise-en-scène* always revolves around the will to power. Prostitute dominatrices dress and behave like doctors or nurses or schoolteachers or sadistic tormentors – in other words, they impersonate figures who wield direct *power* over the subject, especially a moral power. The masochist places himself at the mercy of the woman. In reality, however, the client is often a male of high status, or at least someone with a grandiose idea of himself. It is as if, in sex, the masochistic subject stages his own powerlessness by handing all his power over to the woman. A kind of self-satire. Erotic masochistic domination marks the typical perversion of the dominant class. And indeed, masochists are often proud of their paraphilia, regarding it as something 'sophisticated', a marker of upper-class status. But all this power conferred on the woman rests on a tacit and fundamental assumption: the deep-seated impotence of the woman.

The Masochistic Pique

One of my analysands, a male in his 40s, had begun a relationship with a woman of his age, Giulietta, with whom he had intense and tumultuous coitus, verging on wild amorous passion. Yet, he judged this lover as mean, selfish, uneducated, and shrewish. He therefore began a new relationship, a much more temperate one, with a woman he respected, but did not stop seeing Giulietta. With the woman he admired, things went well, but the enjoyments he experienced with Giulietta were 'something else altogether!'

With Giulietta, at the time, sexual liaisons proceeded as follows: he would ask her to urinate and defecate on him. While she urinated on his face, he would lick her vulva and enjoy sipping her urine or kissing her vulva while she was on her period. After these games, he would have a 'special' coitus with her. Then he would disappear for weeks or months, until the urge to 'be treated like a cesspit' – as he put it – came rushing back. He only felt like doing this with Giulietta; he did not fantasise about such things with other women.

Through his masochistic games, he was exacting revenge on the woman. They were the flip side of the contempt he felt for this partner, who found herself quite thrilled by these games. Just continuing to see her made him feel abject, and the scatological games gave physical form to his humiliation. But his degradation was merely a mirror image of the other; and in time, she came to realise that his request for her to urinate on him was, in fact, a reflexive act of retaliation. She broke off with him, saying: 'You literally treated me like shit!'

Every masochistic game enacts a similar form of retaliation: by submitting to humiliation, the masochist ultimately humiliates the other. There is an implicit misogyny in the masochist. In this sense, masochism is a refined form of sadism – performed with irony through a reversal of roles. At its core, *masochism is usually a protest against* the *alia*. And this protest is instantly self-gratifying, as the subject offers up his own body as a readily available substitute for the original object of humiliation. Masochism is a *do-it-yourself* form of punishing the other, mainly the woman.

The masochist may go so far as to forgo orgasm entirely in order to reach surplus enjoyment. One man, for instance, not only took pleasure in his woman having a lover but also devoted himself to serving the couple as a chauffeur and butler. He would drive them to seaside resorts for romantic weekends from which he was strictly excluded, provide them with money, and rub the lady's feet while she made out with the other man. If the lover was in the mood for his woman one night, he would immediately step aside, offering them the marital bed while he spent the night uncomfortably on the sofa.

Now, the explicit sadistic impulses of masochists usually have male, not female, figures as their object. Psychoanalytic common sense might suggest that the true target of the masochist's hostility is the woman he seeks to be crushed or humiliated by. Instead, the masochist is often a champion of women's rights, and all his resentment is mostly directed at figures of male authority. Thus, when he submits to mistreatment by a woman, he offers his body as a means to see a disappointing (paternal?) male figure subjected to female vengeance, as Reik suggested.

The masochist often delights in fantasies – sometimes enacted – of prostituting his own woman. It is important for the masochist that the prostitute-like behaviour is performed by the woman as an honest woman, by the mother 'as a good mother'.[2] Sacher-Masoch encouraged his wife, Wanda, to seek out lovers by responding to newspaper ads and to prostitute herself for money. 'How delightful – wrote Sacher-Masoch – to *find* in *one's own* respectable, honest and *good wife* a voluptuousness that *must usually* be *sought* among *women* of easy virtue' (*Venus in fur*).[3] Wanda did all this to please her master-slave, but for Masoch, it was a way of giving concrete form to what he believed to be a woman's desire: to have many lovers and to prostitute herself.[4] The masochist sees himself as fulfilling unspeakable female fantasies – and at times, he is not entirely wrong. His manipulation of women is gynophilic, not necessarily hostile.

Watching one's partner offer her body to others is a tragicomic re-enactment of a primal trauma: the scene of betrayal by the mother. Men who like to be cheated on – the 'cuckolds' of porn videos – turn their bitter jealousy into the honey of perversion. I would call it *negative jealousy*.

But his woman's promiscuity is also, paradoxically, a form of revenge against the men who enjoy her favours: he, the masochist, *knows*, while the other *knows not*. He is the director of the spectacle, and the man who, in his dull unawareness, delights in the woman the masochist loves is a pitiable creature, lured in by the cheap bait of the female body. The other man is a puppet in the hands of the 'director'. What matters most to the masochist is that the woman is his accomplice.

Swingers

Among the array of *negative jealousies*, we should also consider the 'lifestyle' or 'swinging' within the partner-swapping community.[5]

For an analysand who took up swinging in his early 50s, the crucial element was not sleeping with the woman of the other couple, but watching his own wife seduce the 'other' man or the 'other' woman and witnessing the sexual play between her and the man or between the two women. For him, it was more about voyeurism than exchange. The point was that he and his wife could no longer have sex without imagining a scenario involving others. The presence of the Alter – man or woman – had become a *sine qua non* for their sexual life as a couple.

But he keeps raising the bar. He encourages his wife to join a swinger couple without him: the only thing he cares about is that she tells him everything afterwards. The woman agrees. But then he raises the bar even higher. A single man is attracted to his wife, so he pushes her to accept a lovers' holiday to the South Seas with him, *as long as she tells him everything*, and maybe even shows him some videos of their sexual encounters. In short, the analysand realises that what he wants is 'a slut'. So much so that … he becomes aroused imagining her falling in love with this new lover.

It should be noted that throughout his life, this man had been by no means passive or submissive; quite the opposite. A talented, audacious entrepreneur, he knew how to give orders and had the makings of a leader. For him, *lifestyle* was the crowning achievement of a successful life.

In Lacanian terminology, we can say that the desire of the subject leans on the desire of the Alter: the object (the woman) only becomes truly desirable when the Alter desires her. And the Alter enjoying her is a source of enjoyment. But on condition that the woman-object remains *one's own.* What excites the swinger is not taking a woman from another, but giving his woman to another, a giving that remains completely under his control. Therefore, the swinger could not bear the thought of his woman having sexual intercourse with another *without his knowledge.* Knowing and seeing is the mark of an inalienable possession. In the absence of such a mark, the masochist may slip into a positive, even destructive jealousy.

The passion of the swinger is a negative jealousy, in that the chronically jealous too are not so much tormented by their woman's or man's infidelity as by *not knowing* what that woman or man is doing with someone else. Both positive and negative jealous types are obsessed with the truth: *knowing* is the real great power they can wield.

Jealousy, in general, is not, as Melanie Klein seems to think, the fear of losing the loved object.[6] Jealousy is not truly 'utilitarian'. In cases of delusional (paranoid) jealousy, the jealous man does not particularly love his woman – what obsesses him is being deceived, *cheated.* Othello never says he fears Desdemona will leave him to live with Cassio; what horrifies him is that *he does not know* and cannot see Desdemona's and Cassio's amorous acts. It is not the fear of abandonment but the loss of knowledge-power over the beloved other that obsesses the jealous person. What gives pleasure to the negative jealous person, the swinger, is precisely seeing the partner's adultery and taking part in it. And indeed, if he discovers that the woman he loves has a relationship that has been kept hidden from him, his negative jealousy instantly becomes extremely positive – he will throw terrible jealousy fits, because the woman has stopped being his accomplice; she has truly *betrayed* him. That is, he suddenly discovers he has no power at all over the other.

The swinging is mostly promoted by the man, although often the woman not only adapts to it but also becomes captivated by the game herself. In some cases, however, it is the woman who imposes swinging, and the man reluctantly follows. One such case is particularly instructive.

A 40-year-old man, a very accomplished engineer, is deeply in love with his wife, whom he considers a goddess, and whom he greatly admires. But for years he has had no desire to have sex with her; their sexual relations are sparse and unsatisfactory, while he has a long string of affairs with young girls of low social and intellectual standing, with whom he repeatedly indulges in intensely erotic, provocative games. It is one of those cases described by Freud (1912d) as 'debasement in erotic life', where a man completely separates love from sexuality. Love within a couple is based on the convergence of two tendencies, tenderness and sensuality, on the same object, but this convergence is not always accomplished. The classic case in Freud's time were men who were impotent with their beloved wives, and who then regularly went to 'release the tension' in brothels. Sexual satisfaction is only possible for them with degraded women. Our engineer is one of these men. The point is that his wife, evidently dissatisfied with her husband's sexual performance, suggested swinging. Obedient to his beloved wife's will, he bowed to her wishes, but every swapping experience was a nightmare for him: he was terribly jealous of his wife in this situation, has no desire to have sex with the woman of the other couple, but did not let his revulsion transpire in front of his wife.

We realise that the wife probably likes the swapping and that she was trying to be sexually unfaithful to her husband while, at the same time, remaining symbolically faithful to him (swinging is like leaving a door open and closed at the same time), but that she is also trying to appear to him as a lowly slut. In short, she seems to be hoping – in vain – that by presenting herself to her husband as a debased sex object, she will arouse his erotic desire for her.

Caesaristic Sexuality

In the film *Take the Money and Run* (1969), we see Woody Allen's character growing up in a grim and violent slum. A frail child, he is often beaten up. They tear his glasses off, throw them to the ground, and trample on them. Accustomed to this relentless mistreatment, the older Woody introduces a twist: the moment he senses an attack coming, he rips off his own glasses and stomps on them himself.

This gag exemplifies what psychoanalysts have termed 'identification with the aggressor',[7] a process Freud described to account for a puzzling phenomenon: neurotics appear to inflict suffering on themselves for no plausible reason, sometimes not even an unconscious one. In the end, he saw the notion of primary masochism – and, in the background, the death drive – as the key to making sense of this enigma.[8] In reality, however, the introduction of radical, non-erotic masochism is a way of reformulating the mystery rather than solving it.

On the way to this conclusion, Freud speculated that many forms of self-inflicted suffering still obey the pleasure principle (*Lustprinzip*), albeit indirectly: by turning the subject from a passive victim into an active agent of pain, they offer a form of consolation, restoring a sense of mastery. Like Allen – who, unable to avoid violence, prefers to inflict it on himself, taking a desperate pride in the act.

Like every perversion, masochism too is a strategy for deriving enjoyment from something that was initially intensely unpleasant. The masochist repeats – in an erotic key – a painful experience.

In sum, what matters most to the masochist is securing mastery not only over the *alia* but, above all, over his own passivity. Like any artist who depicts their own defeat, it is through this active representation of abjection that their control ultimately prevails. Such was the case with the first true best-selling novel of the modern world, Goethe's *The Sorrows of Young Werther.*[9] Here, the author drew inspiration from his own unhappy love affair with a married woman. The difference is that, in real life, Goethe had made a swift exit, whereas in the novel the protagonist, Werther, takes his own life. The author's enjoyment consisted in turning his failure into a supreme defeat, suicide. And in this way, he achieved a literary triumph by representing this supreme defeat.

The reversal of passivity into activity can, however, take on very twisted and sophisticated forms.

A man, Mathieu, has had a double sex life since his youth. He has been married to a woman, with whom he has children, but would occasionally have casual affairs with other women. At the same time, he regularly went looking for young men – and continues to do so even now that he is over 75 – to sodomise. In every city or region where he has lived, he has invariably and quickly found spots where he could find such 'passive' men. His relations with these, mostly young, men were limited to the 'low' sphere, and he rarely established an affectionate relationship with any of them. He says that what is important to him is to make the other person enjoy anally, an experience from which he excludes himself as he abhors being sodomised. Whenever he enters a state of anxiety or depression, he goes in search of men to sodomise.

He believes this passion stems from a scene in his childhood. When he was 5 years old, the doctor prescribed an enema for him, and, like most children, he refused to submit to it. He had to be held still by three adults, and his father eventually managed to insert the pump into his anus. It was in that moment that Mathieu felt the flood of hot water penetrate him and felt an intense enjoyment, similar to what an adult would experience sexually. It therefore became essential for him to make the other enjoy passively while he played the role of the father with the enema. He was the Alter of his male lovers.

In his partners – men who seek only passive sexual encounters with other men – another twisted process unfolds. Based on my clinical experience with this type of man whom I don't label as bisexual, they lead a conventional heterosexual life, often living with a female partner and having children. Yet, from time to time, they feel the need to be sodomised – they point out – by the largest possible penises. They never form a truly affectionate bond with their sodomiser, who is often a casual partner, and sexually they allow him anything except kissing or embracing. Tenderness is entirely excluded from these encounters, which remain strictly genital. They are not particularly attracted to men; they desire women, and some are even womanisers, yet now and then they feel the need to 'play the female'.

It seems to me that this is a case of what I would call the Caesarist complex. When Julius Caesar became the *de facto* emperor of Rome, he was said to be 'every man's woman and every woman's man'.[10] At the time, being sexually active with other men was entirely acceptable, while being passive was seen as utterly contemptible (ancient Romans had no concept of 'homosexuality'). Now, these men who want to be treated as females often have a grandiose self-image, an almost imperial bearing. They want to be everything and anything – both male and female … and more. Usually, however, it is a masochistic enjoyment that guides their 'becoming female'. In fact, they may engage in masochistic games with their female partners. Deep down, they see femininity as something humiliating – being possessed, yielding – and it is precisely this humiliation that they seek in passive sexual relations with men. They play a feminine role because they despise femininity.

Their orgasms are, of course, phallic, so their *special* enjoyment lies entirely in being penetrated. In this sense, 'Caesarist' enjoyment reveals a dimension of female sexuality that women themselves often repress. The act of penetrating a woman is felt as an act of abuse, and it is precisely this abuse that 'Caesarists' take pleasure in – that is, they derive enjoyment from the fact that females like them are 'disrespected', the same as in the past, at a time when the mere fact that unmarried women had sex with men made them unworthy of respect.

Notes

1 See Francis of Assisi (2012), in particular Chapter 8.
2 Deleuze (1971, p. 57).
3 Sacher-Masoch (1999).
4 Wanda von Sacher-Masoch (1990).
5 See Gould (1999). On the French swingers' planet: D. Welzer-Lang (2005).
6 Melanie Klein (1957) says that the origins of jealousy lie in the fear of losing what one has. Jealousy, in short, is summarily reduced to the anguish of losing something.

7 This notion was developed by Ferenczi (1932) and Anna Freud (1936).
8 Freud (1920g).
9 Goethe (2005).
10 Suetonius (2025, par. 52).

Chapter 4

A Case of Masochism

Lorenzo's Impossible Wife

When Lorenzo, a high school teacher, first comes to see me he is 65. Slender and agile, he carries an aura of sarcasm, projecting an attitude he calls '*sprezzatura*' (a studied carelessness and nonchalance). His manner of speaking is histrionic; he clearly wants to impress me. In our sessions, especially during the first year, he puts on a one-man show that expresses a fierce kind of rage.

For decades, his sex life has largely been limited to visiting prostitutes. In the past, he only went with dominatrices. The services he required of them were to be whipped on the buttocks, urinated on, and covered with clothespins all over his body, especially on his nipples and scrotum. As is common with dominatrices, he never engaged in full intercourse with them. Until recently, however, he had also gone to 'regular' prostitutes, with whom he could have penetrative sex – albeit reluctantly – and would usually stop before ejaculating.

Before me, as he endlessly repeats, he has had 25 psychotherapists from various schools. He mocks all of his former psychotherapists. One even gave him a diagnosis: *borderline narcissistic personality*. Consequently, he took to reading books on this syndrome.

'I'm only coming to you because you're an S&M specialist', he tells me. 'Here's what I want: now that I'm 65, I want to experience sacred love, not just profane love'. In other words, he wants a woman to marry him and bear his children. 'I've been with 130 whores in my life, and I've also tried my luck with 130 women who weren't prostitutes, but all of them turned me down'. He dreams of finding a wife who also enjoys sadistic play, someone who will whip him and

DOI: 10.4324/9781003531388-4

urinate on him in bed. He does not want to change what he calls his 'sexual orientation'. He speaks openly about his paraphilia to anyone without the slightest sense of shame.

> Little by little, Lorenzo eventually admits that it is not the women who say 'no' to him, it is he who says 'no' to them. He is afraid of penetrating them. It is a Copernican revolution from his point of view.

Lorenzo has a high opinion of himself as a cultivated man, but at the same time he sees himself as a sorry figure from the poor rural Italian South. The utmost self-idealisation, the utmost self-denigration. And any interpretation of mine, no matter how sharp, will not faze him in the least – he will just say: 'some other psychotherapist already told me this!'

The Analyst Loses His Patience

His sexual-anthropological system gradually takes shape. Lorenzo calls any woman who is already in a relationship with someone else and does not want him a *zoccola* ('slut'). Starting with '*quella zoccola di mia madre*' ('that slut of a mother of mine'). Women are the object of his resentment. There are only two women he does not call 'sluts', and one of them happens to be a prostitute – Lola. Single women, on the other hand, are all held in high regard. Among them, he includes a nun he fell in love with before she took her vows, in addition to a few lady friends who have chosen not to engage in sexual relations with men. As for the latter, they are all qualified as '*coglioni*' (arseholes, jerks). The prototype of the *coglione* is his own father, who left all power to his wife, especially over his children, without any say in the matter. Or men who could not or did not want to procreate; in this sense, he himself belongs to the *coglioni* species.

In this human sea of *coglioni*, a tiny elite of people he respects stand out – among them his former teacher of comic-book art and, more recently, me. At first, his transference towards me is provocative and dismissive; he repeats that I won't be able to give him what he wants either.

There is, however, a turning point.

After skipping sessions for three consecutive weeks, he tells me: 'What's the point of me coming here? You're rather disappointing'. And he starts whining again about his failed relationship with Beatrice a few years earlier. I feel it is time to let my patience run out:

> I'm tired of you showing up here and repeating the same things over and over again, and always in the same terms. You come here and put on a show, just like you do with your schoolgirls, but I'm not one of your students. I find it pretty boring to hear the same drivel again and again. So, either you change your tune or your presence here is useless. If you're just going to come back and tell me for the thousandth time that Beatrice would come on your face when you licked her pussy, then you're better off staying at home. You didn't show up for three weeks, not because of your COVID quarantine, as you claimed, but because you just didn't want to come. The last time I told you that you could have married Lola if you'd wanted to, you were so shocked that … you ran like hell. If you want, you can spend your life stewing in revenge against Beatrice and Barboni. That's your choice, but then there's no point in wasting your time and mine.

I should point out that I often adapt to the language of my analysands.

So, Lorenzo realises that his histrionics do not work with me. Consequently, a strong transference finally begins – one not without its share of adulation. He tells me again and again that after 25 psychotherapists he has finally found 'the smart one', someone who doesn't beat about the bush. For a while, he begins every session with: 'I have been admitted to the court of Sergio Benvenuto!'

At other moments during the analysis, I notice a turning point whenever I lose my patience and give him a good dressing-down. Lorenzo wants me to lay into him. The irate analyst gives him a taste of the father he never had. Lorenzo has an extreme need not for authoritarism but for authoritativeness, what Lacan called 'the paternal metaphor'.

> His transference unfolds as a grand idealisation of me, albeit laced with envy. He dreams of one day becoming a member of my family. For a time, he fantasises about marrying my daughter (whom he believes he once saw standing outside my building).

He despises 'ordinary people', including his fellow teachers. Ordinary people marry, have kids; there's always a son doing drugs, the mother-in-law with Alzheimer's, as the husband ages he gets involved with a much younger woman, and so on and so forth. The bleakness of normality. When I point out to him that his insistent demand for a normal family seems contradictory, since he basically abhors the prospect, he remains impassive: 'Who isn't contradictory?' He is right, of course.

'Ditch Amalia!'

I retrace the family myth that Lorenzo built for himself *via* his mother.

Lorenzo was born in a rural village in southern Italy. That *arsehole of a father of his* counted for nothing – at home his mother was the 'mistress of the household'. According to him, she married his father, though she never loved him, just to have children. Even in her youth, his mother's body slumped slightly to the left – according to her, this was because she had breastfed her younger, heavyset brother. This early maternal burden had curved her 'like a slave'. She lost her first child within a month of birth because, as she said, 'my milk became toxic'. Lorenzo's birth was also difficult – he was born breech. At first, he refused to breastfeed and could have starved to death until the ghost of an aunt 'moved' him so that he could latch onto the nipple. So, has Lorenzo always been *spostato*? In Italian, this means both 'unhinged' and 'displaced', and it also refers to 'a misfit'.

His first four years, he recalls, were idyllic. He was the darling of every woman in the village; he was clasped to their ample bosoms like a treasured jewel. Out of jealousy, his mother took him away to the town of O., ostensibly to be nearer a paediatrician who, she insisted, had to attend to Lorenzo constantly –

always, she claimed, on the brink of death, like her first son. 'I have been *abducted* by my mother ever since', he says. She had no voluptuous breasts to offer him. He diagnoses himself as an uprooted child.

From the age of 11, he has been fascinated with westerns. At this age, the defining *scena-madre* (literally a 'mother scene' in Italian, but also a term from drama denoting a pivotal or climactic moment in a play or film) took place: he was caught by his mother playing in front of the mirror wearing a bandolier like a gunslinger. She slapped him. So, he stopped pretending to be a cowboy and started wearing his mother's clothes in front of the bathroom mirror. Looking at himself in feminine attire, he would become aroused and masturbate. According to him, wearing women's clothing was an act of self-humiliation.

He still often admires himself in the mirror and sees himself *with a beautiful female body.* He sees himself as an attractive woman with a penis and no breasts.

This slap from his mother is the pivotal trauma of his 'sexual orientation': the act that punishes him for using a gun/penis has to be repeated over and over again for him to become sexually aroused. Every morning he wakes up with an erection and imagines variations of the same scene: a beautiful woman – sometimes a nun – punishes him for his erection. She commands him: 'Don't come! Shame on you'. Only occasionally does this arousing scene culminate in masturbation and orgasm.

He had his first girlfriend at the age of 24, in O. Their relationship lasted three years. However, he never had full sexual intercourse with her. In the car, he would perform cunnilingus on her until she had an orgasm. Then she would rub his face and penis with her feet, but he would make her stop just when he was about to come. His mother seemed happy that he had a girlfriend, but then she developed cancer that eventually took her life. Lorenzo is convinced that she 'brought the tumour upon herself' because he was with a girl. After his mother's death, he left the girl.

Around the age of 35, he began a relationship with Amalia and moved in with her at her house in Rome. He appears to have had a normal sexual life with Amalia. She became pregnant and had an abortion. At this point, the second *scena-madre* occurred.

He had gone with Amalia to O., to the house where he had lived as a child, where they had sex – with sadomasochistic foreplay – in his parents' bed. The next morning, as Lorenzo was making coffee for himself and Amalia, the water began to boil, and a sudden spurt shot out – in that instant, he heard his (dead) mother's voice say: 'Ditch Amalia!'

A hallucination? He would obey this maternal command.

From the age of 39 onward, his life revolved around dominatrices. His attempts to seduce non-prostitutes, he claims, always ended in failure. This narrowing of his sex life to 'mistresses' runs parallel to the string of '25 therapists' and the long sequence of failures with the '130 sluts' who rejected him. But at 63, with two women, things took a different turn.

Love Without Sex

At the school where he teaches, he meets Beatrice, a teacher 30 years his junior. He describes her as 'a small, fragile child', flat-chested, like a little girl. As it happens, she has the same scoliosis as his mother – except that she underwent surgery and is now 'bolted'. He would later tell me that when he sees a woman with a limp in the street, he is moved to tears and … 'I feel I want to marry her', he says to himself.

Beatrice falls in love with Lorenzo. She visits him at home once a week, and – on this occasion too – Lorenzo limits himself to cunnilingus, which makes her 'come on my face'. This 'coming on my face' seems to be very important to him. But he does not achieve an erection, and therefore cannot penetrate her. He never progresses to full sexual intercourse with Beatrice: 'I couldn't care less about sliding my dick up and down', he insists. 'Penetration is for brutes'. However, he takes great pleasure in bringing Beatrice to orgasm and asks her to marry him. Beatrice, however, bursts into tears and breaks up with him.

He would later tell me that he dared not have masochistic fantasies with Beatrice, but sadistic ones instead. I suggested to him that perhaps Beatrice was disappointed because she wanted full sexual intercourse. His reply: 'I couldn't fuck her. I wanted to marry her first, in the Vatican, with a bishop officiating, and then make her pregnant … Women today are sluts: they want to fuck before marriage!' Is this him or his mother talking? He repeats that he is a victim of his mother, who has been dead since 1983. He insists on this hyper-protected childhood of his. One day I say to him: 'You're not a victim of your long-dead mother. *You are your mother*!' He is struck dumb by the remark.

His mother gave him an overly prudish upbringing as a child, and his sexual mentality seems stuck in the 1950s. He has had several priests and even a bishop as spiritual advisors. I wonder to what extent he is a believer. 'I believe and I don't believe. I'm undecidable, like Schrödinger's cat in quantum mechanics'.

At the time of Beatrice, there was a fellow teacher at school, Barboni, younger than himself: 'That clown!' They were best friends for years. Months after breaking up with Beatrice, 'the clown' confides to him that he had a fling with Beatrice … (Barboni knew nothing about Lorenzo's relationship with her). Lorenzo tells me again and again that he never believed him, because he considers him impotent – he basically describes him as being like himself. (He assumes that Beatrice has little or no sexual intercourse with her boyfriend. He wants to think of her as chaste, a virgin even.) After this revelation, an overwhelming hatred for his colleague takes hold of him. He has a breakdown. At school, he begins accusing his colleague – without any evidence – of vile acts. For months, he doesn't show up to teach. During this crisis, he would have killed Barboni. I ask him: 'Why would you want to take revenge on Barboni when you're sure he's impotent?' He replies that the unbearable thing is *having told him* he had a fling with Beatrice, *not that he actually had one.*

He brings me a dream:

> I'm in my house in O., which is also the staff room at my current school. It's a parent–teacher meeting. I'm a pupil and a teacher-psychologist is talking to me. Then my mum comes in and starts talking to her while I'm at the other end of the room. I'm scared of what the teacher-psychologist might say to my mother.

He points out that years earlier he had invited Beatrice into that same staff room, where he had asked her to marry him. He gave her a cross as a pendant, even though she was an atheist.

For him, the teacher-psychologist in the dream is Beatrice, and his mother stands between her and him. As with Amalia, years before, the ghost of his mother *does not want him to marry another woman*. Lorenzo constantly denounces his mother's pervasive presence in his life, yet he remains unable to free himself from it.

He had previously brought me a dream in which I appeared:

> I come to your office, but instead of finding you, I'm met by a young woman in trousers, dressed in a yellow-green, 1960s-style outfit. She's taking notes and tells me you're on your way. You arrive, but you're younger, very cheerful, very lively, a whoremonger … Suddenly, I'm on the seafront in O., and I see you. 'What are you doing here?' I ask. You reply that you have to catch a bus and walk away.

The young woman dressed in 1960s attire evokes his adolescence. He dreams of an analyst (me) whom he envies: younger, a ladies' man, with an attractive secretary. He wishes he had known me when he was a teenager. But then, in the dream, I abandon him. It is as if he were saying: 'You left me on my own during my adolescence, when I needed you most!'

He tells me that he lives alone in Rome and has no friends. That he spends his time reading and watching westerns. He has no friends because everyone bores him – they're uncultivated or stupid, basically 'arseholes' or 'sluts'. But delving deeper into his life, a different scenario emerges: in fact, his social life is quite intense; he is seductive with women, and some make it clear to him that they would like a romance with him, but he simply doesn't notice. From here comes the conclusion, which he accepts with difficulty: it is he who rejects the series of women who have openly offered themselves as lovers, not the other way around.

Lorenzo realises that he will never find the sadistic woman he has been looking for. S&M games, he knows full well, are simulations, theatre. For a long time, though, he insists, angrily, that he wants a woman who will agree to marry him.

He has set himself up to enjoy not coitus with a woman, but the denial of coitus by a woman. And when it is a woman asking for sex, the he-as-his-mother rejects her, this time with no pleasure.

A Gunless Man

Is there something psychotic about Lorenzo? Was the fateful voice of his mother ordering him to ditch Amalia a hallucination? The fact is that not all hallucinations are psychotic.

Lorenzo has had at least one other hallucination. In 2007, he went on an organised trip to the United States to visit the iconic sites of the Far West. He saw God in a small town in Nevada. One evening, he went to stand by a graveyard. From this graveyard an enveloping 'something' rose and wrapped him in an embrace, like that of a loving mother. It was his only experience of direct contact with the divine.

The masochistic scene Lorenzo endlessly repeats seems to be the '*mother scene*' from when he was slapped at the age of 11. The S&M rituals are like prolonged repetitions of that slapping in an erotic key.

The young Lorenzo reacted to his punishment for his phallic prowess by dressing up like his mother and masturbating: he combined in his mirror image the female (maternal) body and the phallus. Is the function of this fantasy to attribute a phallus to his mother and to the woman? If this were the case, according to Freud, masochism would be very similar to fetishism: it would consist in attributing a phallus to the woman; without it, the woman would feel humiliated and abused. It is as if the masochist gave all phallic power to the woman, relinquishing his own, his 'guns' in Lorenzo's case. And to do so, he has to play the role of the humiliated and abused in the place of the woman. Hence his female identification. An erotic masochist like him invokes feminine masochism. He plays the masochist the same way a female, according to him, would play the part of a masochist with a man. Revealingly, his ideal woman is the female gunslinger in westerns, the woman on horseback who can shoot like a man.

Lorenzo is dominated by the dictatorship of the maternal Alter. This Alter, a jealous ghost, bars him from what he calls 'sacred love', which means marrying in the Vatican and having children. His mother condemns him only to profane love, to prostitutes.

It turns out that when he was 13 his mother asked her confessor to indicate a prostitute who could initiate her son. After that, she tied a votive bracelet around his wrist dedicated to the Lord with the name 'Lorenzo' inscribed on it. I point out that throughout his life he has done exactly what his mother wanted him to do: '*go with whores*' (which in Italian also means 'fuck up'). And never get married.

He claims he never penetrated Beatrice because he wanted her to marry him first. But what makes him believe that he would have an erection in wedlock? Instead, he delights in licking the vaginas of these women he 'respects', as if wanting to verify, to the point of spasm, that, contrary to appearances, a woman does not have a penis.

'Beatrice came on my face', he repeats, emphasising the squirting of vaginal fluid. An *imago* of an ejaculating vagina? This image actually means he cannot *de facto* give the penis to the woman, but he *must make sure that the woman has it* … a very contorted operation. Having coitus ('sliding up and down') is of no interest to him because his duty is to give the woman phallic potency. Yet this phallic potency in the woman apparently humiliates and devastates him. Hence his resentment against 'all sluts'.

How does this sadomasochistic dialectic relate to the social isolation he complains of? We have said that it is not real: in fact, Lorenzo is 'a very amiable person'. He does not adapt to social relationships, just as he does not adapt to relationships with women: he is limited to either profane love (sadomasochism) or sacred love (a divine marriage). A slip of the tongue in particular is revealing: when he speaks of Beatrice, meaning to refer to her as '*la mia donna*', 'my woman', he says 'Madonna'. He cannot find a middle ground, one that will help to solve the gaping contradictions. For him, someone is either brilliant or pathetic, just as women are either 'sluts' or 'nuns'.

The Saintly Woman and the Whore

I learn that he became infatuated with Beatrice the day after Lola the prostitute told him she was pregnant – another scene that still obsesses him. One day he went to see Lola, and she announced 'I've fallen in love!' – not with him, but with a young Romanian. A month later, she cried out with joy again, so he asked, 'Are you getting married?' To which she replied: 'No, I'm pregnant!' He would repeat these two scenes to me over and over again, as if Lola had fallen in love with him and *he* had made her pregnant. Soon, Lola would give up being an escort and move to Northern Italy to live with her partner and two children, unmarried.

Lorenzo still loves Lola in his own way because 'she's a woman with balls': a gunslinger. For him, women must *have balls.* I remark: 'But if they have balls, they don't need your dick'. On the one hand, we have Lola, whom he admires because she has balls; on the other, little Beatrice, a fragile and crippled woman like his mother, whom he does not penetrate … because he would break her. The drifting of his love from Lola to Beatrice traces a fractured completeness: he has had sex with Lola but never married her (although it is obvious that this is precisely what the Romanian prostitute wanted) and proposed marriage to Beatrice instead of having sex with her.

He had intercourse with Amalia for years, but only because he could stay at her place. Lorenzo says he never loved her and that he was not particularly interested in coitus. It seems that the famous coffee-machine scene took place when he realised that he could love Amalia. In fact, the scene took place after a particularly passionate night of lovemaking.

Lorenzo abhors coitus because he finds it beastly, brutish. 'I respect women too much'. The woman's desire to receive a penis is clearly unacceptable to him. He could love Lola because escorts are not interested in sex: they receive many penises, but none is worth anything to them. 'I could go for months without fucking', Lola said. The woman 'with balls' that he idealises has no need for the male, even when she loves him.

He wonders whether deep down he is homosexual. He tells me that years before he had fallen in love with a non-op trans person, but didn't dare 'suggest' anything to them. He tells me about his fantasy of being penetrated by a woman with a dildo. I remark: 'You definitely don't like men; you like women. But they have to have a penis'. In other words, he is gay with women.

Years before he also wanted to get engaged to a girl, but since he never dared to have intercourse with her, in the end she said to him: 'You're a homosexual priest!'

He tells me about his first sexual intercourse. It was with Amalia, and he was 34: he was able to follow through because the woman was on his lap, so he had the impression that his penis was coming out of her vagina. In short, he had to 'see' that he was the woman and that the woman had a penis. This is what still happens to him today with prostitutes.

I think that Lorenzo always was 'his mother's phallus', and that this prevented him from *having* a penis and using it with women. The following dream seems to confirm this:

> I'm in the house in O., walking towards my room. The same room as the coffee-machine scene … But instead of my bed there's a rattlesnake threatening my sister, who's screaming in terror. My mother comes in, picks up the snake, unfazed, and carries it outside.

I remark that I identify the rattlesnake with him, a 'biting cock'. He agrees. In fact, his sister was a very attractive girl, and he would take her along with him, showing her off as if she were his girlfriend. He desired her.

Here is another dream:

> I'm at an exhibition in a venue where I meet an architect. I talk to him and tell him that an exhibition of his works is being held and that a booklet about them is published every week. That architect was you, Dr Sergio Benvenuto!

He sees me as the prestigious architect who must 'rebuild' him. But he also displays his contempt for me: the fact that he pays me for each session degrades me to the status of a prostitute. His previous analyst once said to him: 'You treat me like one of your whores'. And he was right. As the Italian psychoanalyst Elvio Fachinelli understood, the analyst is often a prostitute for the analysand: a person paid to establish that special erotic relationship known as transference. Which can indeed be compared to the sublime love for a prostitute.

He despairs and says the structure of his desire will never change, and I remark: 'But your desire has changed over time … For example, four years ago, after Lola – your best therapist – you managed to say "I love you" to a woman and to propose marriage to her'.

Lorenzo accepts the idea that Lola had indeed been his analyst: he would go to her not for sex, but to talk at length about himself. And, all considered, he says, Lola cost him even more than I do.

Another dream:

> I'm driving to a villa-sanctuary which is at the top of a hill, travelling along steep roads lined with small exotic-looking lanterns. Beatrice and her father emerge from the villa. Then a religious procession begins, and they join in. Beatrice's face is completely covered in soot, as if she were meant to atone … it looks like she is about to be sent to the stake like a witch.

Beatrice's father is a prominent industrial executive.

I say: 'For you, Beatrice is either divine or satanic. A saint or a witch to be burnt at the stake. But that's an avatar. You're missing the Beatrice who wished to have your penis'. He clearly falls in love with women who belong to the Alter. Beatrice belongs to her father, Lola to her partner, the man who gave her children.

I continue: 'According to you, women are all sluts. The best women are real escorts, like Lola. But if a woman wants to be fucked, she becomes a slut'. I point out to him that both he and Lola wanted marriage: she needed to marry to obtain Italian citizenship, and he wanted to marry because only in this way was he allowed by his mother to have sex. Nevertheless, their wishes did not bring them together.

There is no doubt that he loves women, not mere females. But he cannot tolerate the limits of women; he cannot tolerate the woman as a limit.

As for Barboni, he eventually admits: 'Barboni is my alter ego'. He does not so much envy Barboni because he allegedly had intercourse with Beatrice, while he failed; rather, what is at play here is a reverse identification. This is why he says he is convinced that Barboni is impotent, like himself. But little by little he changes his perspective. He finally says: 'Before, I couldn't believe that Beatrice and Barboni fucked, now I think it's possible'.

He usually refers to Barboni as 'the clown'. Why a clown? Because he has no substance, he is two-dimensional – he is a *semblant*. I say: 'You're the clown, the tissue paper. You think you are getting revenge on him, but you're only getting revenge on yourself. You're perfectly content in your prison in O., the one your mother put you in; otherwise you would have left it. But, unfortunately, this prison doesn't exist. Your defamatory acts of vengeance against Barboni and Beatrice are pure clownery'.

In fact, years earlier, he had tried to slander both.

'You'll End Up Like Don Quixote'

Fragments

As a child, he used to draw scenes from the Wild West, but his mother would tear up his drawings and say, 'You'll end up like Don Quixote'. Even now, his favourite hobby is sketching scenes inspired by the Far West.

He often repeats to me something my 'colleague' Lola once said to him: 'You're not the child of non-love; you're the child of a sick hyper-love'. Simple, but true.

He also talks about his sadistic side. Watching the flagellation in Gibson's film *The Passion of the Christ* gives him pleasure. He identifies simultaneously with the scourged Christ and the flagellators. Watching spaghetti westerns, he enjoys the sadistic scenes involving women.

He always penetrated Lola from behind – he couldn't bring himself to look her in the face because he loved her too much. He says: 'Fucking makes me sick. I don't want to see the face of the woman I love when I'm fucking her'. He finds scenes of sexual intercourse in films repulsive.

Dreams

1 'I'm in my room in O., my bed is there but there's also an extra bed. My mother is lying in my bed and I'm sitting next to it. I put my arms around her and almost pull her out of the bed, but she protests'.
2 'I am in a dormitory with several beds. I'm alone and playing a lonely masochistic game with clothespins. Three students come in and want to occupy the three empty beds. They're accompanied by a little nun in a white dress … I have to compose myself. At one point the nun says: "No, I'm not wearing a chain. I put everything on my vagina"'.

The dormitory in the second dream is a reference to the residence where he lived during his university years.

He wonders whether in the first dream he might have wanted to rape his mother. What is certain is that as an adolescent he never hugged her. In fact, he was extremely aggressive. He shouted constantly at her, and he hit her. Exactly what he does with many of his friends, and sometimes even with me.

He associates the nun's words about 'putting everything on my vagina' with pregnancy. He associates the little nun with Beatrice. I add: 'Yes, but a Beatrice who doesn't fuck, who has taken a vow of chastity'. *Madonna*, in fact.

His mother, he insists, is the primary cause of all his problems. I remark: 'Your mother *ordered* you to go with *sluts*, and you've been obeying her all your life'. And she also ordered him not to love any other woman. But the point is: the mother he lashes out at is his Alter, who is suffocating him. He cannot yet grasp this distinction. He still believes that his real mother, the one who died many years ago, inhabits him.

He says: 'When I'm fucking with a woman, I feel like I'm suffocating … It's like she's sucking me in. I felt the same way with my mother, who also suffocated me'. As a child, he wanted to smash his mother's face into the wall and crush her. And his first girlfriend used to put her feet in his face. 'I wish I was a vibrator women could use to give pleasure to themselves'.

The vagina makes him think of a bloody gash, and he is afraid of becoming violent. His masochism is the other side of his – mostly silent – sadism towards women.

He says: 'I turned Lola, a former escort, into a devoted mother and housewife. And I turned Beatrice, a former angel, into a slut'.

He tells me another dream:

> I'm in a ditch; I'm tying a man's hands and feet. He looks like Ugo Tognazzi. There's also a woman nearby – I think she's Beatrice. I try to tie her up too.

Tognazzi, a popular Italian actor known for his pleasure-loving lifestyle, makes him think of someone who has plenty of sex, who loves the finer things in life … He associates him with Barboni. In the dream, he is basically preventing coitus between Barboni-Tognazzi and Beatrice; he is preventing the sexual encounter that haunts him so terribly.

It seems to me that this unbearable sexual encounter between Beatrice and Barboni cannot exist for Lorenzo because for him to have sexual intercourse with a woman and to be a brutal thug are one and the same thing. And a woman who enjoys orgasms during sexual intercourse is a 'slut'.

'When you risk falling in love with a woman', I tell him, 'you hand her to someone else.' In fact, he handed Lola over to her 'brute' of a man and, effectively, Beatrice to Barboni. He takes pride in having 'found' a partner for Lola, but the idea of having 'given' Beatrice to his alter ego is unthinkable to him.

Woman's Joy

We talk about his sense of loneliness, despite his busy social life. 'Not only am I *alone*, but I do not exist. I have no desires. I don't feel myself. I have had women beat me so that I could feel myself through pain'. I tell him that, quite simply, he has no wish to fuck a woman. He replies: 'I wish a woman would *force* me to fuck her … Then, dominated, I would do it. I set up my own masochistic pantomimes, but I wish a woman would amaze me. Why do women never amaze me?'

I point out to him that if he wants a woman to amaze him, then she won't amaze him at all. It's like the final plot twist in a film: the dramatic turn that surprises us is carefully studied. In other words, the real surprise would be if there were no twist. He wants women to be so intelligent … only to become mere mannequins in his hands. A double bind.

I add: 'In the end, you've succeeded perfectly in life: you've managed to make every woman who wanted to love you leave you. According to the wishes of your …' I didn't add '… mum'.

During one session, he tells me that now he has both 'sex' (another Romanian escort he is seeing) and 'affection' (our sessions). Both of which he *pays for*, he stresses. But there has been an evolution in his sexual encounters with the prostitute. He can now look at her face while fucking her. In other words, the prostitute is gradually starting to resemble a normal woman. Since he has a scientific background, I remind him of what an asymptote is.

A perverse person who seeks analysis is never simply a pervert. The pervert does not want to overcome his perversion because it gives him the very condition of his sexual enjoyment. But analysis becomes possible when someone recognises the high cost of that pleasure. A pervert who seeks analysis is a failed pervert.

I am not indifferent to him. I am touched by his desperate need to be loved – which is really a desperate need to love. What can I give him now that he is 67 years old? An analyst must not desire the good of the analysand, but I share his pessimism.

Besides, he is the type of person who could never accept being 'saved' by an analyst, because that would be tantamount to admitting that the analyst was better than him. Many people who seem to have benefited greatly from analysis never acknowledge it. There is a certain pride in not healing and in proving to the analysts that they are a failure. Lorenzo takes pleasure in repeating '25 psychotherapists have failed with me!' How can I deny him this enjoyment?

My colleagues diagnosed him as having a narcissistic personality. But what does 'narcissistic' mean? There are so many kinds of narcissism. And besides, we all need a certain dose of narcissism. When and how does our narcissism turn against us, contradicting itself?

His narcissism takes the form of pride-and-contempt for others. For the first few months, he was arrogant, displaying a supreme scorn for everyone. Then he entered a more 'depressive position', as Klein would say. The 'pride-and-contempt' shows its reverse side: self-deprecation and admiration for the Alter. The masochistic game is the staging of anti-narcissism: the dominatrix is the 'gunslinger girl' and he's a poor wretch. What in his social life is completely denied through pride-and-contempt reappears as enjoyment in his sexuality. His masochism is entirely a dream of love.

There are only two women he would not use the term 'slut' with: Amalia and Lola. By 'slut' he means any woman who has sex with other men but not with him. A 'slut' is a woman who betrays him with another man. Lola, however, precisely because she went with everyone, remained symbolically faithful to him.

He didn't ask Lola to marry him; like Parsifal, he let the Holy Grail slip away. Only once did he say to her, 'Why don't we get together, you and me?' But she brushed off the suggestion. He could certainly have insisted. Lola would have married him to obtain Italian citizenship and secure a husband with a decent pension. In any case, I believe she had genuine affection for her client.

His love for Lola exploded on the occasions she exclaimed loudly 'I'm in love' and 'I'm pregnant'. The day after this second scene, Lorenzo met Beatrice at school and was instantly love-struck. He realised that he had transferred his love for Lola, the prostitute, to a 'respectable girl', who was clearly not a virgin, but whom he 'thought' was one. It is the classic Catholic overlap between the whore and the saintly woman – Mary Magdalene and Mary the Virgin,[1] the two Marys, or the two faces of Mary.

What makes Lola sublime in his eyes is her being in love and being impregnated by the Alter. He tells me that he gave Beatrice a painting of the marriage of the Virgin Mary and Saint Joseph. I point out that for the Catholic Church there was never a real marriage between Mary and Joseph insofar as they never had sexual intercourse. According to Catholic doctrine, marriage becomes a sacrament only when coitus is consummated between the man and the woman. If he had sex with Beatrice, that would have constituted a marriage in the eyes of the Church. He was not aware of this.

One of his dominatrices had sent him out to buy a pair of shoes; he returned with them and stayed at her house after her 'working hours'. As he watched her, he became aroused and stretched out his hands, for once not thinking of S&M games. But she told him, 'No, you're being punished', reminding him that she was still his 'educator'. She added: 'But if you give me 70 euros, I'll give you a hand job'. He refused, saying: 'I don't want to fuck you. I want to be with you'. And he left.

This 'being with you without fucking you' says a lot about Lorenzo's impasse, which consists of having a woman who will not allow him intercourse, who will be with him as a desirable but forbidden woman.

Experience teaches us that a patient is on the path to terminating analysis when they finally reconcile with their parents, even if they are dead. The parents cease to be objects of hatred and are forgiven; the resentment subsides. The subject separates from childhood once and for all. Something like this is happening to Lorenzo.

We begin to see the image emerge from the lethal puzzle in which Lorenzo is enmeshed. What is it about Lola's two exclamations that so enchant him? He replies: *The woman's joy*. And he recalls several occasions in his life when he witnessed a woman's joy. He remembers one of his would-be wives singing Bob Dylan songs, Beatrice singing her favourite tune, 'Californication' by Red Hot Chili Peppers, and also his first girlfriend singing. He also tells me about a girl he liked and who looked radiant because she was going to become a nun. He felt love shining in her eyes, filling him with admiration. A joy, however, the woman receives not from him, but from the Alter, from pop singers or from God. He seems to fall in love with the woman's love for the Alter, but to him the realm of the Alter seems inaccessible.

Shortly before she died, his mother, such an anxious and hateful woman, had found a kind of serene peace he had never seen in her. 'Before dying, she radiated a certain light'. The same light that those women radiated when they shouted out their love.

'A woman radiates light when in proximity to that limit', I point out to him. To die or love. It was the same light he had seen in that little village in Nevada, which came from the graveyard. I also point out that, to describe his vision in Nevada, he had used the expression 'an enveloping embrace', the same 'enveloping embrace' he attributes to his mother, except that hers had been to suffocate him. The vision fulfilled the mirage of a relationship with his mother that was no longer one of suffocation. It is as if for him the woman becomes adorable when she rejoices in the Alter to the point of death: then the feminine light that dazzles him appears.

He came to me after being humiliated and scarred by the triangle with Beatrice and Barboni. Had it not been for that setback, the consequence of his desire to love a woman, he would never have come. He came at the right time, when he most needed it, although that time was already nearing the final verses of the ballad.

Note

1 Almost everyone believes this, even though in the Gospels Mary Magdalene is by no means a prostitute, but a woman tormented by seven demons, whom Jesus exorcises.

Chapter 5

Cross-Dresser, Trans Person, Transsexual

From Cross-Dresser to Queer

Both DSM psychiatry and psychoanalysis draw a clear distinction between cross-dressing (the updated term for *transvestism*) and *transsexual, transgender*, or *trans person*. The former is classified as a perversion, while the latter is what psychiatry calls *gender dysphoria* – a term strongly criticised by queer culture.[1]

A cross-dresser is a man who not only enjoys dressing as a woman but – an essential trait – takes pleasure in being *mistaken* for one. This does not mean that he is a passive homosexual or that he is 'effeminate', as he would have once been described. He generally leads a full heterosexual life, may be married to a woman and have children, but derives a distinct surplus enjoyment from cross-dressing. Not infrequently, his partner takes part in these cross-dressing 'escapades'. He feels completely masculine, and it is precisely because of this strong sense of his own manhood that he finds the act of appearing as a woman so arousing.

Like most perversions, transvestism is predominantly male. A woman may dress as a man, but this tends not to provoke a particular reaction in others. It might be surprising to discover that someone who seemed to be a man is actually a woman, but this feeling is a far cry from the uncanny sense we still experience when a male gender is revealed behind a female appearance. This is akin to what once happened with

DOI: 10.4324/9781003531388-5

homosexuality: it was always male homosexuality that provoked real scandal. Similarly, F to M cross-dressing is largely neglected. This asymmetry probably stems from the persistent idea in our culture that it is 'normal' for a woman to want to look like, or be, a man, whereas it seems abnormal for a man to want to look like, or be, a woman; we may think of how any woman today can choose to wear either trousers or a skirt as she pleases, but it remains unacceptable for a man to wear a skirt. We can say that the *marked sex* is the male: it is acceptable for a woman to masculinise herself, not for a man to feminise himself.

Essentially, it is as if the cross-dresser sought to denounce the *womanly masquerade*, the art by which women turn themselves into the phallic object of men. Evolutionary biologists struggle to understand why, in our historical tradition, women put so much effort into makeup, jewellery, and colourful clothing to seduce men – as if men had reason to play 'hard to get' and only chose the most beautiful women, whereas in fact the sexes are roughly equal in number. In our culture, the woman seems compelled to compensate for her perceived phallic deficiency through her masquerade, presenting herself to the man as a fetish. Similarly, the cross-dresser offers himself as a pure sexual fetish. This game clearly becomes a satirical parody of femininity in the drag queen, so important for the philosopher Judith Butler.[2]

Instead, the DSM calls gender dysphoric someone who wants to be assigned to a different gender from the one they were assigned at birth. The use of the term *assignment* implies: 'At birth, identifying an infant with male genitalia as male, or one with female genitalia as female is not compulsory'. Being born male or female is no longer a matter of *ascertainment* but of *assignment* – a decision made by adults. And like any decision, it can be arbitrary and, in any case, open to contestation. There is a growing tendency today to downgrade sex, understood as an anatomical and functional reality – namely, the functional complementarity of male and female – in order to make room entirely for *gender*, i.e. a cultural classification. Gender casts such a shadow over sex that it almost makes it disappear.

Earlier psychiatry spoke of 'gender identity' or 'order of gender difference'. These terms, however, imply a kind of indelible mark, given by nature or society or both, whereas the term 'dysphoria' implies something exquisitely affective. The Greek term *dysphoria* means 'excessive pain', from *dys* ('bad') and *phero* ('harbour'), so literally 'dysphoria' means 'to bear something bad'. The term therefore has a strong emotional connotation. It is opposed to 'euphoria' and could be translated as *discontent*. Gender Discontent.

In any case, a gender dysphoric or Trans Person is someone who complains of a discordance between their sexual body and their gender identity. The most common phrase is 'a woman's soul trapped in a man's body' or vice versa. The Trans Person resolutely rejects any assimilation to either the homosexual or the cross-dresser. If they were assigned male at birth and feel they are a woman, they usually reject sexual intercourse with men prior to organic transition (i.e. before genital change) because they would be unable to assume a feminine role in the relationship. If a Trans Person dresses and wears makeup like a woman, they derive no paraphilic pleasure from the masquerade: female clothing is what they feel belongs to them. The same is true in the opposite case.

It is remarkable how gender identity takes up almost all of a Trans Person's mental space, with almost nothing left for object love, that is, attraction to an external person, be it man or woman. The Trans Person is basically not attracted to anyone in particular: their own symbolic inscription in the other Gender is a matter of life and death (as Patricia Gherovici, 2017, puts it); there is simply no time to fall in love with anyone.

It is interesting to note that historically in the Western world, Gender Discontent was much more prevalent among men who wished to become women. In recent years, there has been a reversal, with more women wanting to become men – a shift whose anthropological significance has not yet been fully understood.

A number of psychoanalysts originally regarded Gender Discontent as a form of psychosis: the belief in having a female identity despite having an entirely male body – or vice versa – was seen as a hallucination, not of the senses but of 'feeling as'. Trans people were likened to Chief Justice Daniel Paul Schreber, a famous case of paranoid schizophrenia that Freud and many other psychiatrists and writers commented on.[3] Schreber's delusion revolved around his belief that he was being transformed into a woman by a lustful God who constantly engaged in sexual intercourse with his female self. However, the fundamental difference between a trans delusion such as Schreber's and Gender Discontent lies in the fact that Schreber believed he was truly being turned into a woman through divine miracles, whereas the Trans Person is fully aware that they are not inherently a woman and therefore turns to medicine to make their 'appearance' match their 'being'. This difference between *appearing* as one sex and *being* of the other is not in itself a delusional discourse, because it does not *deny* reality but *exposes* it as mere appearance. Therefore, trans people tend to identify with the realm of the 'oppressed', with those who must achieve emancipation – even though today, in modernised countries, there is full freedom to change one's gender. They expose an unknown Other who has a confused appearance and being in gender.

It must be said that the need for independence from nature expressed by queer culture extends beyond sexuality and encompasses the entire body. First and foremost, surgery is increasingly relied upon to alter significant aspects of the body according to the desires of its bearer. But cinema and literature (especially science fiction) also anticipate this desire/power to completely transform the body. Something that James Cameron's popular *Avatar* films exemplify. In them, a crippled and frail human being, through the use of futuristic technology, completely transforms his body to move around on another planet inhabited by a very different population, where he becomes agile and strong, a leader and hero of its people.

It is commonly said that the difference between sex and gender is that sex is given to us by nature, while gender is a cultural construct. Being male is *sex*; being *macho* is *gender*. Hence the endless, decades-long debate about what proportion of our typically masculine or feminine behaviour is a result of our chromosomal sex and what proportion is a 'social construct'. (A debate that presupposes a clear conceptual separation between the biological and the cultural, between nature and nurture, which I do not believe should be taken for granted.) The approach known as 'constructivism' claims that the characteristics of each gender, purely cultural-historical constructions, are completely divorced from our biological determination. History, not hormones, makes us 'male' or 'female'.

The concept of gender largely swallows up the concept of sex, since being born with a penis or a vagina is no longer sufficient to determine the corresponding gender. What matters is that the physiological characteristic is perceived, accepted, and subsequently registered by those who receive the child. The linear implication between sex and gender is thus further broken down: What marks transgenderness is not the claim to belong to a gender that conflicts with one's biological sex, but rather the claim to belong to a gender other than that *assigned by others.* This is a capital distinction.

Three Ways of Being 'Trans'

Psychiatric clinical practice notes a statistically significant difference between those who experience gender dysphoria or discontent early in life (during childhood) and those who encounter it later on, in adolescence or adulthood.

The born male who wants to be female from childhood will almost always be attracted only to males (*androphilia*) after puberty, but will never identify as gay. Similarly, the born female who wants to be male from childhood will be attracted only to women (*gynephilia*) and will never identify as a lesbian. In adolescence, both will seek surgical or hormonal correction of their biological sex and, once they have done so, rarely regret it.

The story is quite different for those who become Trans Persons during puberty. First of all, most late-onset Trans Persons are male. This preponderance of males among 'tardy' Trans Persons should make us sit up and take notice, especially considering that transvestism too is a largely male phenomenon. In most cases of late-onset male transgender subjects, neither the person nor their parents recall any signs of this discontent in childhood – it simply did not exist at the time. Often, these late-onset Trans Persons engage in typical cross-dressing practices, deriving sexual pleasure from being mistaken for women, which aligns them closely with paraphilic transvestites. Furthermore, they engage in something that early-onset Trans Person individuals never do: *autogynephilia*.[4] That is, they experience intense sexual arousal when imagining themselves as women, wearing women's clothing, or looking at themselves in the mirror in such attire. Even more noteworthy is that late-onset male-born Trans Persons, even after undergoing organic transition, are predominantly gynephilic – that is, they are attracted to women or to other M to F Trans Person individuals who, like them, did not transition until adolescence. We could say that they identify deeply with their sexual object: the woman.

A high percentage of adult late-onset trans men live with or are married to individuals born female. Many of them self-identify as lesbians after surgical sex reassignment. We can say that they become the gender to which they are attracted. It is similar to what happens to some women who regard themselves as highly attractive: during sexual intercourse, at the moment of orgasm, they fantasise that they are the man penetrating them.

In essence, it is as if late-onset Trans Persons remained fundamentally cis-heterosexual, even if that heterosexuality is interpreted as homosexuality.

The generic term *transgender*, therefore, brings together two very different *subjective structures*, as these are understood in psychoanalysis. It would seem that the authentic Trans Persons are those who are transgender from childhood, while those who become transgender in adolescence lie somewhere between transgenderism and paraphilia. In short, tardive transgenders could be considered a type of cross-dresser. To distinguish them, I propose calling them *Imaginary Transgenders*, even when they undergo surgical transition. On the other hand, I would restore to early-onset Trans Persons the name that best describes them: Transsexuals – even when they do not undergo an anatomical transition.

A distinction must, however, be made between both the Imaginary Transgender and the Transsexual, and the Cross-Dresser as described above. Some Cross-Dressers may have sex with men, but only when they are in female clothing. In short, submitting to anal penetration is part of their feminine masquerade. Usually, the cross-dresser who prostitutes himself tends to play the active male role in sexual intercourse, as this is what the client usually wants. But the cross-dresser experiences intense sexual arousal when, and sometimes *only* when, he is dressed as a woman. In other words, the Cross-Dressed person can have sexual intercourse with a man in order to *resemble a woman* in a peak of verisimilitude, not in order to *feel like a woman*.

The film by François Ozon, *Une nouvelle amie*,[5] gives us a psychiatrically impeccable portrayal of a paraphilic cross-dresser. David is a widower who, with the complicity of a friend, enjoys dressing up as a woman and being taken for one. But he is not sexually attracted to men. In a cinema, for example, a man sits next to him in the dark and sensually fondles his legs; David takes obvious pleasure in this. But later, he points out that he was by no means attracted to the man and only delighted in being taken for a woman and treated as one. The cross-dresser does not reciprocate the man's erotic desire for him.

Some argue that cross-dressing may, in certain cases, represent the first step in a progression toward Gender Discontent: when it is no longer a matter of occasionally wearing women's clothing but rather of wanting to *always* be dressed as a woman. As we have seen, however, this progression from cross-dressing to Gender Discontent only occurs when the latter arises during adolescence. In other words, in the case of Imaginary Transgenders.

'Trans' for Psychoanalysis

The Freudian descriptive model can help us to distinguish between these subjectivities much more accurately. Psychoanalysis makes some important distinctions.

(A) It distinguishes between 'object-libido' – the erotic desire for an object external to the subject – and something quite

> paradoxical that Freud calls 'ego-libido'. Ego-libido means not that the ego as a whole, but rather its image, becomes the object of sexual attraction. This is what happens in sexual narcissism: a subject sexually enjoys their own image, particularly in the mirror. Autogynephilia (mentioned above) is evidently a form of sexual narcissism.

Autogynephilia represents a space where ego-libido and object-libido intersect: the sexual object of the cross-dresser or Imaginary Transgender is female (belonging to the opposite sex), but the subject derives a surplus of sexual pleasure insofar as the 'hetero' arousing object is the feminine image of their own body. At this point, another analytical concept begins to operate:

> (B) The Ideal-Ego, which Jacques Lacan distinguished from the Ego-Ideal.[6] The Ideal-Ego refers to the ideal mirror image of the self that each of us has. In the Cross-Dressed or autogynephilic ('Imaginary Transgender') it seems clear to me that the Ideal-Ego has a female form, but this Ideal-Ego is also the object of erotic arousal. Those with a reversed gender sexually desire women because the female form remains their ideal form; except that they derive pleasure not only from an object with a female form, but also from themselves as participants in that ideal female form. It is as if they were making love to two women at the same time: one with an idealised female form, and themselves as shaped by their own feminine ideal. Hence, their declaring themselves lesbians.

In the case of real Trans Persons – those who have been transgender since early childhood, and whom I have proposed calling Transsexual – the structure seems to me to be quite different. If they are born male, it is not because femininity is their Ideal-Ego that they feel female; after all, not even masculinity is their ideal object. Rather, what is feminine is their *Ego-Ideal*, as Lacan would say, distinct from the Ideal-Ego. In other words, they are eager to occupy the symbolic position of 'female', much like someone who is determined, at all costs, to occupy the position of

'Prime Minister' or 'President'. We could say that the office of Prime Minister represents their Ego-Ideal, while their Ideal-Ego might lie more in *performing the role of Prime Minister* than in *being* the Prime Minister. These Transsexuals do not accept that their anatomical masculinity negates their symbolic femininity ('my female soul'). It is not their *performing the role of a woman* or *appearing as a woman* that arouses them; if anything, they may be aroused by a man insofar as they, as subjects, *are women*. The point, however, is that they are not aroused *like* a woman, as would be the case for a completely cis-woman; they are aroused *because of* their *being* a woman, which distinguishes them from born females. Their Ego-Ideal, therefore, is not a libidinal object; it is desexualised. However, unlike cis women, the male object ideality is not truly sexualised. We can say that in M to F trans people, it is their *being a woman* that is idealised. In a certain sense, hetero trans people have an autoerotic sexuality. In short, I don't think trans people really become the other gender, given that cis individuals are polarised on the other sex object, while trans individuals are polarised on their own gender.

This does not detract from the fact that men and women – even without gender reassignment issues – very often self-eroticise; they enjoy seeing or 'feeling' their male or female forms. But this narcissistic attraction to one's own sexed body is not to be confused with the distinctly erotic excitement of autogynephilia or autoandrophilia, where the attraction to one's own forms takes on a distinctly sexual quality. When this happens, the subject is already on a path that is likely to lead to homosexuality.

On the basis of these considerations – which psychoanalytic categories help to make manifest – so-called Gender Discontent should be divided into two entirely distinct configurations, which in turn are connected – through permutations – to the perversion of cross-dressing.

Let us take the case of a male-born subject. We would have the following coordinates (where F stands for Feminine or Female):

Born Male

Table 5.1 ASSIGNED MALE The Trans Diagram

Psychotic Pole	Neurotic Pole	Perverse Pole	
"Transexual"	"Imaginary Transgender"	"Cross-dresser"	*Proposed Name*
Early childhood	Adolescence, adulthood	Adolescence, adulthood	*Onset*
***	F form	Man's gaze	*Sexual Object*
Ego-ideal: being F	Ideal ego: F form	Being the F ideal of the other	*Ideal*
Symbolic narcissism	Imaginary narcissistic	Transgressive	*Libido*
Androphile woman	Gynephile Man	Actor (who masks him/herself)	*Identification to*
Ego receives it	Ego lacks it	Ego pretends its lack	*Phallus*
Being (a woman)	Act (as a woman)	To pretend (to be a woman)	*Intentionality*

What we have called *poles* correspond to the three major structures that psychoanalysis has isolated and which are designated by three subjective and not necessarily psychopathological groups: psychosis, neurosis, and perversion. We can say that while psychosis and neurosis are a 'loss of reality', perversion is rather a 'denial of reality'.

In *psychosis*, the most characteristic loss of reality is delusion: I take things that are not real to be real. In the case we have referred to as transsexualism, there is no delusion, but there is still a relationship with the reality of one's own body, albeit in the form of an obstacle. One's body is experienced as belonging to the *other* gender.

In *neurosis*, the loss of reality arises from the predominance of the imaginary dimension in real life. In the case we have referred to as 'Imaginary Transgender': 'I know that in reality I am a heterosexual male, but my desire to be a woman prevails. I am what I wish to be; I have no desire to be what I am'.

In *perversion*, what predominates is a fictional denial of reality, not an exclusion of it. In the case of cross-dressing, a man who is and identifies as a man presents himself to others as a woman and takes pleasure in this misperception. Today, authentic female transvestism does not really exist, as any woman can now dress in men's clothing, whereas the reverse is not the case – it is normal for women to wear trousers, not for men to wear skirts.

According to psychoanalysis, at least five elements need to be clarified in order to determine a sexual position:

- the object of erotic attraction,
- its relationship to the ideal,
- with what or with whom the subject identifies,
- the type of libido at play,
- the position of the subject in relation to the phallus.

I have also added the entry 'intentionality', a term by which I mean a fundamental relationship of the subject to being, doing, and appearing.

Regarding the *sexual* object, it is not the same in the Transsexual, the Imaginary Transgender and the Cross-Dressed.

The Transsexual (psychotic pole) is convinced that they are a heterosexual woman, so the man – and the phallus he bears – *has to be* their object of sexual desire. However, as we have seen, their relationship to the *phallus* is not the same as that of a cis-woman. In Transsexuals, we notice a relative indifference to the sexual object.

The Imaginary Transgender (neurotic pole) is aroused by the female body form both in themself and in their partner; this form implies the *lack of the phallus* both in themself and in their partner.

The Cross-Dressed (perverse pole) is instead aroused by the gaze of the other, who *does not look at him as the bearer of a phallus* but as being without a *phallus.*

As regards identification, it is evident that the Transsexual identifies with the heterosexual androphile Woman (with an upper-case W). What distinguishes them from a normal woman is their male biological reality, which is removed (often physically) by the predominance of their Ego-Ideal: being a woman.

The Imaginary Transgender, a structurally neurotic personality (even when they do not complain of neurotic symptoms), identifies instead with the heterosexual gynophile male; however, their object of attraction is the female form, admired both in themself and the other. What distinguishes them from a normal male is their Ideal-Ego, which is the feminine *form*. Whereas for the normal male, the female form, even if idealised, represents the erotic object.

The Cross-Dressed, as perverse, identifies neither with the female nor with the male, but with an actor in a costume. In ancient Greece, in ancient Rome, and in Elizabethan times, the most popular actors were those who dressed as women to play female roles. The erotic object of the Cross-Dressed is therefore the gaze of the audience, i.e. the fact that others see him as a woman and believe him to be one. In this case, therefore, we should assume a libido that is different from both object-libido (which invests in an external object) and narcissistic libido (which invests in the image of the ego itself): I would propose the term *transgressive libido.* By this term, I mean the fact that the subject is aroused by something that should not be done, that is forbidden: the act of transgressing this norm provides a special pleasure. In the case of transvestism, appearing as a woman is a transgression because the social norm demands that if you are physiologically a man, you are required to dress and behave as one. Let us bear in mind that Joan of Arc was condemned to the stake for a specific crime: dressing as a man. In the Middle Ages, disguise was a serious crime punishable by death. Pleasure is all in appearing.

We have also seen the different positions with respect to the phallus. To recapitulate: the Transsexual M to F aims at receiving the phallus. Whereas the cis-heterosexual man seeks the phallus by giving it to the woman, the Imaginary Transgender enjoys the lack of a phallus, which takes no part in the game; in short, they practice an a-phallic sexuality. As for the Cross-Dressed, he finds pleasure in the fact that he has a phallus but is concealing it: being perceived by others as a being without a phallus is exactly what he wishes to achieve and which provides him with a surplus enjoyment.

As we can see, the psychoanalytic approach describes three different subjective structures, whereas the DSM describes only two. But it sees two, not because it is authentically a-theoretical as it claims. In fact, the DSM follows an implicit theory: that what matters whenever someone has problems with their 'gender' is the incongruence between their physiological sex (although it calls it 'assigned gender') and the gender that the subject lays claim to. For the DSM, this incongruence is all the disorder amounts to, which is evidently a theoretical choice like any other. Whereas what emerges as decisive in psychoanalysis is something observed across all three positions (the psychotic, the neurotic, and the perverse): the mode of sexual enjoyment. These modes of enjoyment all involve a disconnection from one's anatomical sex, though at different levels.

We can say that for all three, there is a disconnection from the fact of their sex, male or female. However, whereas for what we have called the Transsexual, the fact is disconnected from *being* (a woman), for the Imaginary Transgender, it is a matter of *playing the role of* (a woman), and for the Cross-Dressed, it is about *appearing as* (a woman). The same applies, of course, to subjects who are 'assigned' female at birth.

All in all, according to today's dominant narrative, sexuality – particularly as gender, and perhaps as sex too – is more and more something *chosen*. In a way, Simone de Beauvoir's famous statement – 'One is not born, but rather becomes, a woman' – has been taken literally.[7] Which was ultimately a variation of Nietzsche's 'become who you are'. The Trans Person too wants to become what they are. It is true that the vast majority of women and men end up 'choosing' – or having imposed on them – their 'assigned' sex, that is, their biological sex.

But then why classify transsexualism as a disorder? Mainstream psychiatry is caught in a contradiction. On the one hand, the liberal narrative frames gender as a matter of individual choice. On the other hand, there is the functionalist and naturalist narrative that we have already outlined. Is gender a choice or an optimal adaptive function?

The trans position has become claim-based, in the sense that the Trans Person increasingly demands that the state provide for their gender reassignment. In other words, the Alter is expected to perform an act perceived as a matter of justice. Not appearing as *their own* gender (the one they wish to transition to) is decried in the same way as one might decry an inefficient health service or their taxes being too high. The Alter, in the form of the state – or, more broadly, cis society – is the subject of a constant, nagging question, as if gender reassignment were its responsibility: 'The Alter messed up by assigning me to one gender; now it must see to it that I am incorporated into the other'.

Notes

1 On the basic distinction between transvestitism and transgenderism: Stoller (1968); Ambrosio (2009). Among the psychoanalytic approaches to transgenders: Millot (1991); Cavanagh (2017); Lemma (2018, 2022); Gherovici (2017, 2024); Gherovici and Steinkoler (2022).
2 Butler (1990).
3 Schreber (2000); Freud (1911c).
4 This term was introduced by the sexologist Ray Blanchard. See Bailey (2003).
5 Based on the short story 'The New Girl Friend' (Rendell, 1985).
6 Lacan (1975, Chapters X–XI).
7 de Beauvoir (1997).

Chapter 6

Paedophilia

In recent decades, it has become increasingly difficult to discuss paedophilia in a detached and objective manner, even within scientific publications. Today, paedophilia – even paedophilic desire that does not lead to acts – arouses a sense of horror that did not exist until a few decades ago.

Also, many psychoanalysts are not able to conceal the revulsion they feel towards their paedophile patients, and this subliminally perceived revulsion, of course, triggers a persecutory negative transference in the patient towards the therapist. It is as if these therapists, when they write a case report, were implicitly saying to their readers: 'Don't think that because I treat paedophiles, I sympathise with them! I find them just as repulsive as you do'. In fact, psychotherapy for paedophiles is often ordered by the courts.

In particular, many psychotherapists are horrified by the fact that such patients usually don't display any sense of guilt. On the contrary, they often claim 'I am no paedophile', and swear that they genuinely love children, especially those who appear unhappy or distressed. Most paedophiles are neither rapists nor violent sadists; instead, they are men or women who 'understand' children and are able to win them over through words and acts of kindness, thereby often eliciting an acquiescent response from them. In fact, only a fraction of paedophile acts come to our attention, because children usually don't disclose what some adults have done to them, in part because there was a form of complicity on their part.

In short, most paedophiles – some of whom also express themselves in publications[1] – feel unfairly persecuted. And this is what

DOI: 10.4324/9781003531388-6

distinguishes them from other paraphiliacs: usually a masochist or a cross-dresser or an exhibitionist admits the strangeness and even the illegitimacy of his acts, more rarely so the paedophile.

Many paedophiles equate themselves with gay males. They believe that paedophilia will undergo a historical process similar to the social acceptance of homosexuality: over time, society will come to recognise that they *love* children. They say that their feelings are rooted in 'the laws of the heart'.

In the face of this self-absolution on the part of their paedophile analysands, some analysts react like the average person: they are appalled. They see their role as guiding the paedophile to acknowledge one or more of the following: (1) their guilt in the face of moral law, (2) that they are unwell, or (3) both. Psychotherapy then becomes a soft form of torture, because it essentially aims to extract a *full confession* – in this case not of the act itself, which paedophiles usually admit, but of their own moral guilt.

In analytical practice, it is common to encounter analysands, mostly women, who complain of having been sexually exploited by adults – usually their father, other close relatives, or family friends. Paedophilia is often intertwined with incest. And, of course, the suspicion of incestuous paedophilia lies at the very foundation of the invention of psychoanalysis. Thus, addressing paedophilia unavoidably brings us to the subject of familial incest and the origins of psychoanalysis.[2]

Jean Laplanche's theory, which revived Freud's early 'seduction theory', originally advanced to explain the symptoms of hysteria, enjoyed a certain success among psychoanalysts.[3] Freud initially believed that female patients had been sexually 'molested' as children by adult family members, particularly male ones. He later came to think that these attentions were primarily fantasies of desire on the part of the young girls (without excluding that in fact sometimes this desire had been 'fulfilled' by the concerned adult). Laplanche, however, argued that the human unconscious in general – not just that of girls who would grow up to become neurotic – is based not so much on intentional seduction of children by adults, but rather on a kind of cryptic seduction. Adults transmit 'enigmatic messages' to children, prompting them to ask

'What does the other want from me?' All children, without exception, must 'translate' this ambiguous adult sexuality into their own language, and this translation will lay the first stones from which the unconscious is built. Put differently, it is a sort of generalised paedophilia on the part of adults that makes us human. According to a psychoanalyst, having an unconscious is the defining feature of being human. In Laplanche's view, it is paedophilia that builds our psyche.

This theory of Laplanche, despite its unlikeliness, has convinced many analysts because it satisfies the presupposition Laplanche himself calls 'the primacy of the other' in the formation of one's psyche.[4] A certain philosophy states that almost everything we are does not come from genes nor from our body, but rather it is a sort of imprinting of our early social relations in childhood. Our deep desires are transplanted from outside; the others' desire constitutes our own. This is also called the *relational* view in psychoanalysis.

Discovery of Paedophilia

The horror surrounding paedophilia is a relatively recent phenomenon in our Judaeo-Christian and hyper-industrialised world. Research conducted in both the US and France reveals that the terms *paedophile* and *pédophile* rarely appeared in newspapers such as *The New York Times* and *Le Monde* before 1996.[5]

Since the 1990s, paedophilia has become a subject of alarm for the general public, despite the fact that reports of CSA (Child Sexual Abuse) have shown a steady decline in industrialised countries.

In the 1990s, allegations of childhood sexual abuse against close relatives – fathers, mothers, grandparents, aunts, uncles … – reached almost epidemic proportions. Many adults 'remembered' incidents from their childhood and accused family members, often even taking legal action.

In many films and stories at the turn of the millennium, when an adult character displayed signs of mental distress or imbalance, CSA was almost always found to be the cause. In American studies and lectures on famous writers or artists, biographers nearly always managed to trace the origin of these authors' personal struggles – and their inspiration too? – to some form of CSA. Over time, however, this trend began to wane.

In the 1980s, the trial of members of the McMartin family, who ran a preschool in Manhattan Beach, California, caused a public outcry in the US. The investigation and trial lasted seven years (from 1983 to 1990) and was the longest and most expensive criminal trial in American history. The McMartins were accused of sexually abusing 360 children in their care as part of satanic rituals. In the end, all the defendants were acquitted.[6] During those years, there were various reports of satanic rituals involving underage victims, and today historians speak of the *day-care sex-abuse hysteria*.

In the 1990s, allegations of ritual mutilation of humans, rape and murder of children, of drinking of their blood, and cannibalism – very often the agents were the teachers – spread throughout the US.[7]

The *Boston Globe*'s 2002 campaign on the various cases of paedophilia involving Catholic priests and the cover-up by the church hierarchies of the Archdiocese of Boston, and the subsequent proliferation of similar campaigns across the United States, is widely known. And we might ask why such an investigation was not conducted 20 or 30 years earlier. In fact, the crusade against paedophilia – both involving priests and family members – originated primarily in the United States in the 1990s, and only later spread to Europe and other countries.

Today, everybody knows about the conspiracy group QAnon, which believes in the existence of a network led by Democratic Party officials that allegedly has two primary goals: the installation of socialism in the United States and paedophilia.

In 2016, an urban legend began to gain traction: that a certain pizzeria in Washington, DC, was the centre of a child trafficking ring for paedophiles, with Hillary Clinton at its head ('Pizzagate'). In December 2016, a certain Edgar Maddison Welch stormed into the pizzeria and fired at the locked door of a presumed den of paedophiles.

Kidnappers and murderers whose victims are minors are often classified as paedophiles, even though this does not necessarily imply the presence of paedophilic paraphilia. For example, Marc

Dutroux is commonly referred to as a paedophile. Dutroux, a 39-year-old Belgian, kidnapped six girls between 1995 and 1996, aged between 8 and 19, raped and tortured them, and killed four – either by starving them to death or burying them alive. According to experts, what mattered to Dutroux was not the fact that some of the victims were children, but that they were all female. His case, therefore, falls more accurately under the category of homicidal sadism.[8]

I will not dwell on the distinction between paedophilia (sexual acts with pre-pubescent children) and pederasty (sexual acts with adolescents). Adolescent sexual development is a continuous process, and a 14- or 15-year-old is fundamentally different from a 12-year-old. In some American states, so-called 'Romeo and Juliet' laws allow sexual acts between minors or with minors under specific conditions, while in others, any sexual activity between minors is prohibited. The patchwork of regulations and exceptions concerning teenagers in various state legislations highlights that sex with pubescent minors does not carry the same implications as sex with pre-pubescent children.

Among Catholics, until the 1990s, parents who sent their children to clergy-run schools had to take into account the fact that their male children would be the object of attention of some priests, while female children would be the object of attention of some nuns. It was part of the experiences a boy and a girl had to have in life, like, for males, going with prostitutes, serving in the army, or having at least one physical fight with a peer.

The play *Doubt: A Parable* by John Patrick Shanley[9] is set in a Catholic school in the Bronx (New York) in 1964. A nun becomes convinced that a parish priest, a charismatic preacher, is involved in an inappropriate relationship with a barely pubescent boy from a humble social background. But she has no proof. She speaks to the boy's mother to warn her of the danger, but the mother makes it clear that it's none of her business and that she is actually quite happy that a priest has taken her son, an isolated little boy, to heart. The mother's reaction was typical of the time.

In that period, therefore, any episodes that involved male children with paedophiles were considered to be 'grown-up son things', maturing experiences. In 1979, the famous French child psychoanalyst and educationalist Françoise Dolto,[10] very popular with the general public, gave an interview – for which she was heavily criticised only posthumously – in which she debunked the fear of paedophiles. Dolto also gave the example of teenagers in Rio de Janeiro who had managed to survive and become mature, despite having been involved with paedophiles. The basic idea was again that pederasty (not paedophilia, which Dolto herself condemned) was something a young person might experience.

An Unclear Desire

When medical sexology appeared with Krafft-Ebing and other sexologists of the 19th century, paedophilia did not hold the place it occupies in contemporary culture. It was not a major focus of medical or pedagogical concern. Instead, the primary deviations identified at the time were homosexuality and masturbation, particularly in children – behaviours that official psychiatry no longer considers disorders.[11] Freud, who discussed incest, fetishism, homosexuality, sadism, masochism, and impotence, never mentioned paedophilia.

The question arises as to why the sense of horror – and therefore the particular clinical interest – in paedophilia only began around the 1990s. From then onward, the principle of what I would call *puer sacer*, the sacred and thus untouchable child, took hold. Adults, including parents, were no longer allowed to touch children physically, whether to hit them or to caress them sensually. Today, even the classic slap occasionally delivered to children is considered 'child abuse' and is legally prohibited. Kissing, caressing, hugging – once considered normal gestures between adults and children – today are suspected of being signs of paedophilia. And indeed, it is difficult to draw a clear line at which a caress or an embrace takes on an erotic meaning and turns into 'abuse'.

The prevailing view is that an act constitutes paedophilia if it involves the genitals of either the child or the adult, or both. The genitals are the boundary that, if crossed, however slightly, triggers the offence. But we know that there are many other ways of arousing sexual feelings in children without touching their genitals. For example, if a man shows his erection to a child from a distance, is this a paedophile act? What if a couple has coitus while a child is allowed to watch? It is extremely difficult to determine at what point erotic provocation begins for a child.

Some believe that paedophilia is essentially an adult's sexual desire for a child. If a man or woman undresses in front of a child, there would be nothing wrong as long as *they do not derive pleasure from exposing themselves to the child.* But if they enjoy doing so, then yes, the act is perverse. But how can we distinguish so precisely between an erotic act that happens casually before a child and one performed deliberately to affect the child? Laplanche's revival of the theory of seduction is based essentially on this irreducible ambiguity of what 'seduction' is for a child.

Psychoanalysis, with its stress on unconscious desires, makes the very concept of 'erotic desire' extremely uncertain and volatile. For example, a woman with a number of psychiatric problems states that her mother personally washed her entire body, including her intimate parts, almost every day from early childhood until the age of 26. Can we consider this an incestuous and paedophilic relationship when her daughter was a child? In such cases, we can at best speak of palaeo-paedophilia and proto-incest, because paedophilic and incestuous relationships require a clear separation between the parties involved, whereas here we are at a symbiotic mother–daughter entanglement.[12]

Today, *paedophilic desire* is always execrated, even when the paedophile does not engage in paedophilic acts.[13] It is a desire that is subject to criminal prosecution, a little like heresy was centuries ago: someone could be brought before a court for heresy even if they had not actually written or said anything heretical, merely *thinking heretically* was a crime.

One of my analysands, a woman, used to spend a few days a month at her father's place after her parents separated when she was 5 years old. On these occasions she would sleep in her father's bed and would, so she says, take off all her clothes. Her father would stroke her back, her legs, and sometimes even her buttocks. A habit that ceased when the girl reached puberty. The analysand cannot remember her father going any further than that, but there is always this suspicion that repression intervened to separate the event from its memory. Is fondling a very young daughter's naked buttocks in bed a paedophilic act?

The very notion of paedophilic desire is problematic.

It is important to note that the philosophy of the *puer sacer* does not censor child sexuality when it takes place between children. Child masturbation is no longer frowned upon, and adults look upon 'playing doctor' with some indulgence. Until a few decades ago, however, sexual games between children were severely punished. The opposite of what is the case today was true at the time: sex between children was not tolerated, though they were readily given into the hands of paedophile priests or relatives.

Some are surprised by this horror of paedophilia a century after Freud described child sexuality: 'How can anyone continue to deny that a great many children are titillated by sexual games, also with adults?' According to some intellectuals, the criminalisation of all forms of paedophilia is a cultural 'reaction' against a revolutionary vision that acknowledges child sexuality. Instead, I tend to think that the taboo of paedophilia derives precisely from Freud's 'discovery' of child sexuality.

Before that, no importance was attached to the sexual games that adults might engage in with children because it was believed that sexuality had no meaning for children, that for them their genitals were organs like any other.[14] Significantly, parents often stop playing sexual games with their sons or daughters only when they enter puberty. Today, on the other hand, precisely because we recognise that children have sexual emotions quite similar to those of adults, we take it for granted that adult erotic displays can have an important effect on them. What is unacceptable today is not the fact that the adult man uses the child merely to express his own adult sexuality, but the fact that the adult uses the child's sexuality to satisfy his own. For example, a child is shocked by an erect penis rubbing against them not because they 'don't understand' what the penis signifies, but because they understand it all too well.

Before the 1990s, the wind was blowing in the opposite direction, especially in Europe. Those were the years of the 'sexual revolution', the ideas of Wilhelm Reich and other prophets of liberation from all sexual taboos, which led to the creation of a movement to legitimise paedophilia, one that was particularly vigorous in France.

In 1976, René Schérer and Guy Hocquenghem, two well-known far-left homosexual intellectuals, co-edited an issue of the important journal *Recherches* on the theme of childhood and education, where child sexuality, even with adults, was exalted.[15] The project was endorsed by eminent academics, including Michel Foucault. In 1977, Pascal Bruckner and Alain Finkielkraut, in the essay 'Le Nouveau désordre amoureux' ('The New Chaos of Love'), defended a book in praise of paedophilia by Tony Duvert.

In 1978, as a guest on a television programme alongside Guy Hocquenghem, Foucault denounced the legal framework that 'aims to protect children by entrusting them to psychoanalytic knowledge' and denies the existence of childhood sexual desire, positing sexuality in adults as dangerous. At the time, this campaign did not provoke any particular outcry.

Après-Coup Traumas

We take it for granted that all paedophilic experiences are traumatic for a child. They often are, but not always. Analysands seem to react very differently to the paedophilic events they have encountered.

We accept the fact that certain traumas are an integral part of the psychic development of every human being. Weaning from the mother's breast the first days of school or other separations from the parents are traumas for many children. Puberty is traumatic, and entering working life can also be. The experience of divorce is certainly traumatic for the children of separating parents, as is infertility or menopause for a woman, and impotence due to old age for a man. In many societies, including our own until not so long ago, young males must undergo extremely harsh experiences in order to 'become men'. One need only think of the various *rites of passage* into adulthood in many cultures, rites that we often find excessive and cruel.[16] Compulsory military service for men has been maintained for so long in many countries because it was a way to separate young men from their mothers' skirts through the trauma of the draft. A life without trauma would be a fake life. This is the paradox of human existence: on the one hand, it always tends to avoid trauma, but it is only through trauma that a person truly comes into the world. *Life is risky* because trauma can debilitate a person, but the absence of trauma can be no less crippling.

In order to condemn an experience with a paedophile, therefore, it is not enough to say that it is traumatic. Something more than trauma is required. So, many studies try to quantify the damage that a paedophilic experience can cause to a child.

In this regard, we can refer to the passionate dispute between CSA experts in the US over what is known as *the Rind et al. controversy*. This debate – which unfolded both in scientific publications and in the media – arose in 1998 following research by psychologist Bruce Rind and his colleagues.[17] Their study cast doubt on whether childhood experiences of sex with adults caused permanent psychological damage that persisted into adulthood. The debate caused such an uproar that even the US Congress stepped in to condemn the study – a truly unprecedented intervention in American legislative history.[18] In fact, it is an axiom of liberal democracy that politics should never intervene in scientific controversies. I bring it up here to emphasise that there is no universal consensus among experts about the psychic effects of early sexual experiences with adults.

Empirical research into the effects of CSA is difficult to conduct because so many people who have undergone the attentions of paedophiles as children do not report it and, above all, because each case is different. Paedophilia is condemned not because we have overwhelming evidence that it is always a severe traumatic experience, but because it clashes with the ethical framework of our time, which increasingly prescribes chastity between adults and children. Very often, epidemiological studies are only props to support a purely moral stance.

In psychoanalysis, when discussing the traumatic effects of paedophilia, we cannot avoid the concept of *nachträglich, après-coup* in French, *afterwardness*.[19] Avoiding a complex disquisition of what *après-coup* consists of, we will say that an experience in childhood may not have a traumatic effect immediately, but only much later, for example, in adulthood, because of a recent event that resembles the initial one, but which is not traumatic in itself. In other words, the meaning of a later event makes the earlier one traumatic. To illustrate this in the case of paedophilia, I will refer to a 2018 François Ozon film, *Grâce à Dieu* ('By the Grace of God').

The film is a faithful dramatisation of a real-life event; it uses the real names of the main characters. Three former French Boy Scouts reunite as adults to bring to justice a priest who abused them as children. They also press charges against the Archbishop of Lyon for covering up the paedophile priest for years and continuing to entrust him with children despite knowing about his tendencies. In real life, the two priests were convicted, but the criminal proceedings are still ongoing. The film follows the story mainly from the point of view of the adults who were abused as children.

Now, it is striking that the initial reaction of two of the protagonists when they are reminded of the paedophile priest is one of indifference. They say to themselves, 'It's all water under the bridge; I'd almost forgotten all about it'. But gradually they begin to feel increasingly marked by those childhood events, developing a passionate, obstinate response to the experience and demanding justice. Two of them are by no means fragile individuals and seem to be fully integrated into normal adult life – the third experiences seizures that resemble epilepsy, though it is difficult to establish a link with the abuse. So, was there trauma or not? As the film unfolds, we begin to sense that if there was a trauma it occurred *après-coup*.

As children, the victims were able to respond to the priest's abuse in various psychic ways, but what matters is that their experiences were later reinscribed when the events entered another register – that of the law. I do not refer here to criminal law, but to the law as justice beyond mere legality. Following Lacan, I call this the law of the Alter. It is neither the law of the state nor the 'law of the heart', to which the paedophile often appeals – 'I love children; I don't want to harm them'. It is a law that psychoanalysis itself struggles to articulate, because it refers to something that is neither a private, personal norm nor a written law of the state in which a person lives. It is within the perspective of this law of the Alter that the protagonists of *Grâce à Dieu* come to feel they have been traumatised. So, it is not the trauma suffered by the real child that counts in order to legitimise the laws against paedophilia, but it is the law that requires adults to be chaste with children that creates the trauma.

Ferenczi's Confusion of Tongues

The most widely quoted psychoanalytic paper on the subject is by Sandor Ferenczi, 'Confusion of Tongues Between Adults and the Child'.[20] It seems that Ferenczi himself was a victim of paedophilic harassment as a child. In any event, this 1932 paper focuses on the following idea: the child sometimes expresses tenderness towards an adult that is tinged with eroticism, but the adult then misunderstands this tenderness, interpreting it as a request for sexual, or even genital, love, and proceeds to the act.

But this confusion of languages between adults and children – and often between adults themselves – also occurs in the opposite direction. I think many adults have experienced this: in certain cases, after showing kind and affectionate attention to a child, the child 'misunderstands' and falls in love with the adult, more or less literally. In many cases, children 'take action' towards the adults, but, of course, unless they are paedophiles, the adults do not play along.

One of my analysands firmly believes that he first fell in love, in the adult sense of the term, at the age of 12, with a man of 30. During a summer holiday, this man had taken a special interest in the child's intelligence and perspicacity, had often taken him along and praised his talents to his friends – without, according to the analysand, this ever leading to the slightest 'ambiguous' approach. The boy masturbated and had already had his first ejaculation, but knew nothing about the dynamics of sex. The fact is that he declared to his relatives that he had fallen in love with the man and, returning home, experienced the typical pangs of separation from a lover that he would later experience as an adult. He remembers having fantasies of situations very close to sexual acts. Anyway, this child had a heterosexual adult development.

Receiving special attention from an adult is an important experience for a child; it often arouses a sense of pride in them, which can take on clear sexual overtones.

It is by no means true that children only know the language of tenderness with adults; they often also know the crude language of sexuality, all the more so today, when they are bombarded by explicitly sexual images in the media (which even appears to be contributing to a trend towards an earlier onset of menstruation in girls in the West).

The reverse of what Ferenczi says is described in Thomas Vinterberg's 2012 film *The Hunt*. Lucas is a kindergarten teacher in a small town in Denmark. A 5-year-old girl becomes attached to him because of the special kindness Lucas has shown her. One day, the girl slips a small metal heart into his coat pocket and kisses him on the lips, but he gently rebuffs her. Offended, she tells a teacher that she has seen Lucas's erect penis. It doesn't take long for the village to become convinced that Lucas is a paedophile. He is reported to the authorities, and his family is entirely ostracised by the community. The child later tries to retract her accusations, but it's too late. 'The poor girl is merely trying to suppress the trauma she endured', they say. Although the court eventually establishes Lucas's innocence, the shadow of paedophilia will continue to hang over him.

I mentioned that the perverse act in general transforms the dramatised repetition of an original trauma, which is usually a trauma of humiliation or exclusion, into an instrument of enjoyment – or rather, of plus-enjoyment. This thesis aligns well with paedophilia, assuming it is true that many paedophiles have themselves been victims of paedophiles.[21] They repeat the experience they encountered passively, but this time playing the active role. They are said to 'identify with the aggressor', in the sense that they emulate the aggressor in order to relive the same traumatic experience with the roles reversed.

As with all paraphilias in general, paedophiles too have a double knowledge. On the one hand, they know that childhood sexual emotions, which certainly exist, do not lead to genital engagement, because this would go beyond the child's ability to dominate a genital emotion. But, on the other hand, they possess another knowledge, one of desire, according to which children are almost adult partners capable of responding to adult genitality. They are split: on the one hand, paedophiles know that they are dealing with mere children; on the other hand, they think that children would appreciate a genital sexual exchange.

So, even if the original experience of being molested by an adult did not involve any enjoyment or at most, involved an extremely guilty pleasure, the paedophile repeats this original experience on the assumption that the child will derive enjoyment from his attentions. If the child does not play along and objects, a paedophile will think he has made a mistake in his seductive approach, that the child has fallen victim to a misunderstanding.

But why do paedophiles desire children and not exclusively adult men or women? I say 'not exclusively' because paedophiles often have a sex life with adults as well. Not every paedophile was sexually abused by an adult as a child, so the repetition of the trauma with them in the active position is not enough to explain their attraction to pre-pubescent children. We need an additional hypothesis.

I have previously suggested that, not coincidentally, ancient male pederasty, which was directed at male ephebes (never females), was a consequence of the impossibility of valuing the female sexual object. The Greek woman was basically despised by the free man, so that even if the man was heterosexual and enjoyed coitus with women, a mature male as an *erastes* found a plus-enjoyment, an extra-ordinary pleasure, in loving and sodomising young boys. The *eromenoi*, the paramours – never slaves, always young men predominantly from the higher social ranks – stood in for women as idealised objects of desire, given that women were not considered idealisable.[22] From this perspective, the driving force behind pederasty is misogyny: the more misogynistic a society, the more women are despised, the more likely it is that forms of pederasty will flourish among men.

Even today, deep down, many men wish that women did not have an explicit sexual desire, that they did not aspire to receive the penis. But this is difficult to maintain, especially in a culture like ours where female sexuality is blazoned by all kinds of media. Hence, a substantial rejection of women by the paedophile.

I wonder, then, whether the paedophile's choice is not related to a catastrophic relationship with a woman, towards whom the paedophile has accumulated resentment and disappointment. The child takes on the 'angelic' qualities of the woman of medieval courtly love, *fin'amor*: candour, goodness, innocence, and the rounded forms that recall those of women. The child is loved – even platonically; there are platonic paedophiles – as a female deprived of her degraded lust.

Notes

1 For example, NAMBLA (North American Man/Boy Love Association) and HeartProgress in the United States, or Vereniging Martijn in the Netherlands. In the United States, pro-paedophile groups such as the René Guyon Society have existed since the 1960s. These organisations typically advocate for the legalisation of minors' consent to sexual activity. However, in most countries today, the minor's consent to an intimate relationship with an adult is not considered a valid basis for decriminalising the adult.
2 Among the psychoanalytic contributions to paedophilia: Gosselin (1992); Arundale (1999); Meyer (2004); André and Gosselin (2008); Schinaia (2010); Socarides and Loeb (2019).
3 Laplanche (1989); Laplanche and Pontalis (1968).
4 Laplanche (1989).
5 Neuilly and Zgoba (2006).
6 Eberle and Eberle (1993).
7 Wright (1994).
8 Magnée (2005).
9 Shanley (2005). The author also directed the 2008 film adaptation of his play.
10 Dolto (1979).
11 See Roudinesco (2009).
12 The idea of a symbiotic link, especially between a mother and her child, was developed by José Bleger and W.R. Bion. See Bleger (2012); Eekhoff (2022).
13 See Jahnke, Imhoff and Hoyer (2015).
14 For an in-depth exploration of this topic, see Ariès (1962).
15 The text of the English translation can be found online: https://homintern.soy/issues/11-9-20/comingandgoingtogether.html
16 Among the many examples is the frightening (to us) ritual initiation of young males among the Simbari people of the south-eastern highlands of Papua New Guinea. See Bull (1997).
17 Rind et al. (1998).

18 See Baird (2002).
19 On the Freudian concept of *nachträglich, afterwards*, see: Laplanche (2017); Benvenuto (2018a).
20 Ferenczi (1932).
21 According to some inquiries, around 30% of child abusers have experienced sex abuse in their childhood (Hall and Hall, 2007).
22 On Ancient pederasty see: Lear and Cantarella (2008), Lear (2014).

References

Ambrosio, G., ed. (2009). *Transvestism, Transsexualism in the Psychoanalytic Dimension*. London: Routledge.
American Psychiatric Association (2022). *DSM-5-TR. Diagnostic and Statistical Manual of Mental Disorders, 5th Edition Text Revision*. Washington, DC: American Psychiatric Association.
André, S., and Gosselin, G. (2008). *Qu'est-ce que la pédophilie?* Waterloo: Éditions Luc Pire.
Ariès, P. (1962). *Centuries of Childhood: A Social History of Family Life*. New York: Knopf Doubleday Publishing Group.
Arundale, J. (1999). Notes on a case of paedophilia. In: S. Ruszczynski and S. Johnson (Eds.). *Psychoanalytic Psychotherapy in the Kleinian Tradition*. London: Routledge.
Austin, J. (1962). How to Do Things with Words. In: J. O. Urmson (Ed.). *The William James Lectures delivered at Harvard University in 1955*. Oxford: Clarendon Press.
Bailey, M. (2003). *The Man Who Would Be Queen*. Washington, DC: Joseph Henry Press.
Baird, B. N. (2002). Politics, operant conditioning, Galileo, and the American Psychological Association's response to Rind *et al.*, *The American Psychologist*, *57* (3), 189–192.
Ballard, J. G. (1973). *Crash*. London: Jonathan Cape.
Bentham, J. (1789). *An Introduction to the Principles of Morals and Legislation*. In: J. H. Burns and H. L. A. Hart (Eds.). London: Clarendon Press, 1970.
Benvenuto, S. (2016). *What are Perversions?* London: Karnac.
Benvenuto, S. (2018a). The Après-Coup, après coup: Concerning Jean Laplanche Problématiques VI. L'Après-Coup, *Language and*

Psychoanalysis, 7 (2), 72–87. Available at: www.academia.edu/38022201/Language_and_Psychoanalysis_Volume_7_Issue_2_2018_

Binet, A. (1887). Le fétichisme dans l'amour. *Revue Philosophique, 24.*

Binet, A. (1888). *Études de psychologie expérimentale: le fétichisme dans l'amour.* Paris: Doin.

Bleger, J. (2012). *Symbiosis and Ambiguity.* London: Routledge.

Bruckner, P., & Finkielkraut, A. (1977). *Le Nouveau désordre amoureux.* Paris: Seuil.

Bull, G. E. (1997). A re-interpretation of a male initiation ritual: Back to Freud via Lacan, *Journal of European Psychoanalysis, 3–4.* Available at: www.psychomedia.it/jep/number3-4/bull.htm

Butler, J. (1990). *Gender Trouble: Feminism and the Subversion of Identity.* London: Routledge.

Cavanagh, S. L. (2017). Transpsychoanalytics, *Transgender Studies Quarterly, 4*, 326–357.

Clavreul, J. (1967). Le couple pervers. In: P. Aulagnier-Spairani, J. Clavreul, F. Perrier, G. Rosolato, and J.-P. Valabrega, *Le désir et la perversion* (pp. 91–126). Paris: Seuil.

Collodi, C. (2000). *The Adventures of Pinocchio* (A. Lawson Lucas, Trans.). Oxford University Press. (Original work published 1883).

Cortina, A. (2017). *Aporofobia, el rechazo al pobre.* Barcelona: Paidós.

Critelli, J. W., and Bivona, J. M. (2008). Women's erotic rape fantasies: an evaluation of theory and research, *J Sex Res., 45*(1), 57–70.

de Beauvoir, S. (1997). *The Second Sex.* London: Vintage Classics.

Deleuze, G. (1971). *Sacher-Masoch: An Interpretation.* London: Faber & Faber.

Deleuze, G., and Guattari, F. (1972). *Anti-Oedipus.* (R. Hurley, M. Seem, and H. R. Lane, Trans). London and New York: Continuum, 2004.

Deutsch, H. (1944). *The Psychology of Women: A Psychoanalytic Interpretation.* Volume *1.* New York: Grune & Stratton.

Deutsch, H. (1945). *The Psychology of Women: A Psychoanalytic Interpretation. Volume 2: Motherhood.* New York: Grune & Stratton.

Dolto, F. (1979). Conversations avec Gisèle Halimi. *Choisir la cause des femmes, 44.*

Dostoyevsky, F. (1866). *Crime and Punishment* (C. Garnett, Trans.). wikisource.

Eberle, P., and Eberle, S. (1993). *The Abuse of Innocence: The McMartin Preschool Trial.* Buffalo, NY: Prometheus Books.

Eekhoff, J. K. (2022). *Bion and Primitive Mental States: Trauma and the Symbiotic Link* (The Routledge Wilfred R. Bion Studies Book Series). London: Routledge.

Ellis, H. (1897). *Studies in the Psychology of Sex: Sexual Inversion.* San Francisco: University Press of the Pacific, 2001.

Ferenczi, S. (1932). Sprachverwirrung zwischen den Erwachsenen und dem Kind. English translation, The confusion of tongues between adults and the child: the language of tenderness and of passion. In M. Balint (Ed.). *International Journal of Psychoanalysis, 30*(4), 1949. Available at: www.sas.upenn.edu/~cavitch/pdf-library/Ferenczi_Confusion.pdf, accessed 6 January 2025.

Francis of Assisi (XIIIth Century) (2012) *The Little Flowers (Fioretti)*, ebook. London: limovia.net.

Freud, A. (1936). *The Writings of Anna Freud. Vol. 2. Ego and the Mechanisms of Defense.* Revised ed. Trans. Cecil Baines. New York: International Universities Press, 1966.

Freud, S. (1905d), *Three Essays on the Theory of Sexuality. Standard Edition*, vol. *7*, 130–244. London: Hogarth.

Freud, S. (1911c). *Psycho-Analytic Notes on an Autobiographical Account of a Case of Paranoia (Dementia Paranoides). Standard Edition*, vol. *12*, 1–83. London: Hogarth.

Freud, S. (1912d). *On the Universal Tendency to Debasement in the Sphere of Love (Contributions to the Psychology of Love, II). Standard Edition*, vol. *11*, 177–189.

Freud, S. (1915c). *Instincts and Their Vicissitudes. Standard Edition*, vol. *14*, 109–140. London: Hogarth.

Freud, S. (1920a). *The Psychogenesis of a Case of Homosexuality in a Woman. Standard Edition*, vol. *18*, 145–161. London: Hogarth.

Freud, S. (1920g). *Beyond the Pleasure Principle. Standard Edition*, vol. *18*, 1–63. London: Hogarth.

Freud, S. (1924c). *The Economic Problem of Masochism. Standard Edition*, vol. *19*, 155–171. London: Hogarth.

Freud, S. (1927e). *Fetishism. Standard Edition*, vol. *21*, 147–157. London: Hogarth.

Gherovici, P. (2017). *Transgender Psychoanalysis: A Lacanian Perspective on Sexual Difference.* London: Routledge.

Gherovici, P. (2024). Gender transition between life and death, *Studies in Gender and Sexuality, 25* (2).

Gherovici, P., and Steinkoler, M. (2022). *Psychoanalysis, Gender, and Sexualities: From Feminism to Trans**. London: Routledge.

Giuttari, M. (2006). *Il mostro. Anatomia di un'indagine.* Milano: Rizzoli.

Goethe, J. W. von. (2005). *The Sorrows of Young Werther* (B. Pike, Trans.). Modern Library. (Original work published 1774).

Gosselin, G. (1992). *La pédophilie: analyse psychanalytique de la structure perverse (préface de Serge André)*. Charleroi: Éditions médicales et paramédicales de Charleroi.

Gould, T. (1999). *The Lifestyle: A Look at the Erotic Rites of Swingers.* Vintage Canada.

Greenacre, P. (1959). On focal symbiosis. In: L. Jessner and E. Pavenstedt (Eds.), *Dynamic Psychopathology in Childhood* (pp. 243–256). New York: Grune & Stratton.

Hall, Ryan C. W., and Hall, Richard C. W. (2007). A profile of paedophilia: Definition, characteristics of offenders, recidivism, treatment outcomes, and forensic issues, *Mayo Clinic Proceeding*, *82* (4), 457–471.

Hirschfeld, M. (1910). *The Transvestites: The Erotic Drive to Cross-Dress* (M. A. Lombardi-Nash, Trans.). Amherst, NY: Prometheus, 1991.

Hirschfeld, M. (1914). *Die Homosexualität des Mannes und des Weibes.* Berlin: Marcus.

Hocquenghem, G., & Schérer, R. (eds.). (1976). *Recherches*, no. 22: *Co-ire. Album systématique de l'enfance.* Paris: CERFI.

Jahnke, S., Imhoff, R., and Hoyer, J. (2015). Stigmatization of people with paedophilia: Two comparative surveys, *Archives of Sexual Behaviour*, *44* (1), 21–34.

Kant, I. (1788). *Critique of Practical Reason* (M. J. Gregor, Trans.). Cambridge: Cambridge University Press, 2015.

Karras, R. (2005). *Sexuality in Medieval Europe.* London: Routledge.

Kernberg, O., and Yeomans, F. (2013). Borderline personality disorder, bipolar disorder, depression, attention deficit/hyperactivity disorder, and narcissistic personality disorder: practical differential diagnosis, *Bulletin of the Menninger Clinic*, *77*, 1–22.

Klein, M. (1957). *Envy and Gratitude.* London: Tavistock.

Klossowski, P. (1967). *Sade My Neighbor.* Evanston, IL: Northwestern University Press, 1991.

Krafft-Ebing, R. von (1893). *Psychopathia sexualis: The Case Histories* (D. Falls, Ed.). Chicago: University of Chicago Press, 1997.

Lacan, J. (1975). *The Seminar of Jacques Lacan: Book 1: Freud's Papers on Technique 1953–1954* (J.-A. Miller, Ed.). Cambridge: Cambridge University Press, 1988.

Lacan, J. (1989). *Kant with Sade.* Available at: www.scribd.com/document/513843934/Lacan-Jacques-Kant-With-Sade-1989-51-October-55

Lanteri-Laura, G. (1979). *Lecture des perversions. Histoire de leur appropriation médicale.* Paris: Masson.

Laplanche, J. (1989). *New Foundations for Psychoanalysis.* Oxford: Blackwell.

Laplanche J. (2017). *Après-coup*. New York: The unconscious in translation.

Laplanche, J., and Pontalis, J.-B. (1968). Fantasy and the origins of sexuality. *International Journal of Psycho-Analysis, 49*, 1–18.

Lear, A. (2014). Ancient Pederasty: An Introduction. In: T. K. Hubbard (Ed.), *A Companion to Greek and Roman Sexualities.* Oxford, UK: Blackwell, 102–127.

Lear, A., and Cantarella, E. (2008). *Images of Ancient Greek Pederasty: Boys Were Their Gods.* London: Routledge.

Lemma, A. (2018). Trans-itory identities: some psychoanalytic reflections on transgender identities. *The International Journal of Psychoanalysis, 99* (5).

Lemma, A. (2022). *Transgender Identities. A Contemporary Introduction.* London: Routledge.

Lykins, A. D., and Cantor, J. M. (2013). Vorarephilia: a case study in masochism and erotic consumption. *Archives of Sexual Behaviour, 43* (1).

Magnée, X. (2005). *Marc Dutroux, un pervers isolé?.* Paris: Calmann-Lévy.

Malabou, C. (2022). *Pleasure Erased: The Clitoris Unthought.* Cambridge, UK: Polity Press.

Meyer, L. (2004). Paedophilia: its metapsychology and place in contemporary culture. Paper presented to 43rd International Psychoanalytical Association Congress, March 2004, New Orleans.

Millot, C. (1991). *Horsexe: Essay on Transsexuality.* New York: Autonomedia.

Mills, D. (1993). The lady is a trampler; '50 Ft. woman' fans crave that touch of style, *Washington Post*, 11 December 1993, C1.

Moll, A. (1893). *Les perversions de l'instinct génital. Étude sur l'inversion sexuelle basée sur les documents officiels.* Paris: G. Carré.

Money, J. (1988). *Gay, Straight, and In-Between: The Sexology of Erotic Orientation.* New York: Oxford University Press.

Neuilly, M.-A., and Zgoba, K. (2006). Assessing the possibility of a paedophilia panic and contagion effect between France and the United States, *Victims & Offenders, 1* (3), 225–254.

Pinker, S. (2003). *The Blank Slate: The Modern Denial of Human Nature.* London: Penguin.

Réage, P. (1967). *Story of O.* New York: Grove.

Reik, T. (1953). *Masochism in Modern Man.* New York: Farrar & Rinehart.

Rendell, R. (1985). *The New Girl Friend and Other Stories.* London: Hutchinson.

Ressler, R. K., Burgess, A. W., and Douglas, J. E. (1988). *Sexual Homicide: Patterns and Motives.* New York: Lexington Books.

Rind, B., Tromovitch, P., and Bauserman, R. (1998). A meta-analytic examination of assumed properties of child sexual abuse using college samples (PDF), *Psychological Bulletin, 124* (1), 22–53.

Riviere, J. (1929). Womanliness as a masquerade, *International Journal of Psycho-Analysis*, *9*, 303–313.

Roudinesco, E. (2009). *Our Dark Side: A History of Perversion*. Cambridge, UK: Polity.

Sacher-Masoch, L. von (1999). Venus in Furs. In: G. Deleuze and L. von Sacher-Masoch, *Masochism*. Princeton: Zone Books.

Sacher-Masoch, W. von (1990). *The Confessions of Wanda Von Sacher-Masoch*. San Francisco, CA: Re/Search Publications.

Schinaia, C. (2010). *Psychoanalysis and Paedophilia*. London: Routledge.

Schreber, D. P. (2000). *Memoirs of My Nervous Illness* (I. Macalpine and R. A. Hunter, Trans. and Eds.). New York: New York Review Books.

Sehgal, A. (2018). *Sadism. Psychoanalytic Developmental Perspectives.* London: Routledge.

Shanley, J. P. (2005). *Doubt: A Parable*. New York: Theatre Communications Group.

Socarides, C. W., and Loeb, L. R. (2019). *The Mind of the Paedophile: Psychoanalytic Perspectives.* London: Routledge.

Sofra, X. (2020). The dark reflection of sadism within the brilliance of the narcissistic persona, *Health*, *12* (9).

Solum, L. (2005). Legal theory lexicon: Legitimacy. Available at https://legaltheorylexicon.com/2005/06/legal_theory_le_2-2/

Stekel, W. (1930). *Sexual Aberrations: The Phenomenon of Fetishism in Relation to Sex*. New York: Liveright.

Stoller, R. (1968). *Sex and Gender. The Development of Masculinity and Femininity.* London: Routledge.

Stoller, R. J. (1975). *Perversion. The Erotic Form of Hatred.* New York: Pantheon.

Suetonius (2025). *The Lives of the Caesars*, par.52. London: Penguin.

Sugden, P. (1995). *The Complete History of Jack the Ripper*. New York: Carroll & Graf.

Todd, E. (2023). *Lineages of the Feminine: An Outline of the History of Women* (A. Brown, Trans.) Cambridge, UK: Wiley, Polity Press.

Welzer-Lang, D. (2005). *La planète échangiste.* Paris: Payot.

Wordsworth, W. (1807). My heart leaps up. Available at: https://internetpoem.com/william-wordsworth/my-heart-leaps-up-when-i-behold-poem/

World Health Organization (2018). *International Classification of Diseases, 11th Revision*. Geneva, CH: WHO Press.

Wright, L. (1994). *Remembering Satan*. New York: Vintage.

Suggested Reading

Readers who want to explore the psychoanalytic approach to perversions further may consult the following texts, presented in chronological order. These works can be regarded as the foundational readings in English for approaching perversions.

Freud, S. (1919e). *A Child is being Beaten: A Contribution to the Study of the Origin of Sexual Perversions. Standard Edition*, vol. *17*, 175–204. London: Hogarth.

Freud, S. (1940e [1938]). *Splitting of the Ego in the Process of Defence. Standard Edition*, vol. *23*, 271–277.

Khan, M. M. R. (1979). *Alienation in Perversions.* London: Hogarth.

Stoller, R. (1975). *Perversion. The Erotic Form of Hatred.* New York: Pantheon.

Swales, S. S. (2012). *Perversion: A Lacanian Psychoanalytic Approach to the Subject.* London: Routledge/Taylor & Francis Group.

Index

Note: Page numbers followed by "n" refer to notes.

For Product Safety Concerns and Information please contact our EU
representative GPSR@taylorandfrancis.com
Taylor & Francis Verlag GmbH, Kaufingerstraße 24, 80331 München, Germany

www.ingramcontent.com/pod-product-compliance
Ingram Content Group UK Ltd.
Pitfield, Milton Keynes, MK11 3LW, UK
UKHW020731261026
476920UK00014B/95
* 9 7 8 1 0 3 2 8 5 5 2 8 8 *